Bedpans
to
Boardrooms

By
Sarah Jane Butfield

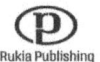
Rukia Publishing

The Nomadic Nurse Series
Book 2

Copyright

©2016/2017 Sarah Jane Butfield

Cover design The Black Rose

Photography by Nigel Butfield

First eBook and paperback editions February 2017

ISBN- 13 - 978-1542625265

ISBN -10 - 1542625262

The people and events in this book are portrayed as perceived and experienced by Sarah Jane Butfield. The moral right of the author has been asserted. All rights reserved.

No part of this book may be reproduced, stored in a retrieval system or transmitted without written permission of the publisher.

Dedication

I would like to dedicate this book to everyone who works within the aged care sector. It is an often misunderstood and undervalued area of healthcare service provision which provides care for our elderly, often vulnerable, population. It also supports younger people trying to achieve a fulfilling life who face the challenges of living with long term chronic disease or disability.

Every person in the aged care sector from management and nursing to care and ancillary staff plays a crucial part in the provision of quality led care.

Thank you to everyone who works in, and supports, aged care residents.

Acknowledgements

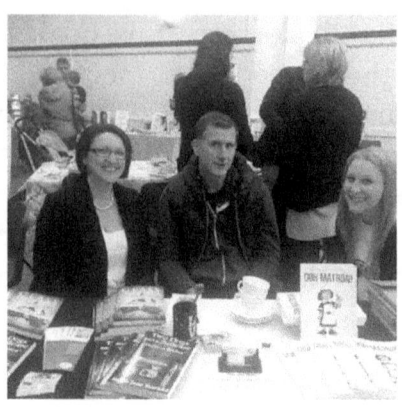

Sarah Jane with her husband Nigel and eldest daughter Samantha at the Llandeilo Book Fair, April 2016

To my husband Nigel, and our beautiful, growing family for their support and continued belief in me and my writing.

I would also like to thank my fellow Wales based authors for their support and encouragement at the Llandeilo Literary Festival led by Christoph Fischer and at the Tenby & Narberth Book Fairs led by Judith Barrow. The support of local authors, and readers, attending these events, is a vital part of the author support network and I am proud to be a part of these talented groups.

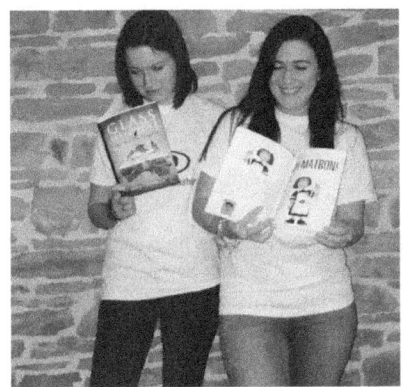

Molly and Jaime preparing for the Tenby Book Fair, September 2016

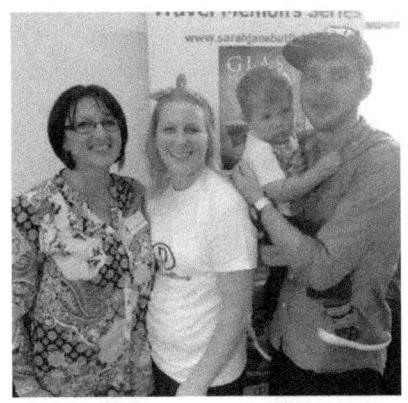

Sarah Jane, Samantha and Robert with grandson Shane at Tenby Book Fair

Catch up on this series so far

*****Award Winning Nurse Memoir*****

The Nomadic Nurse Series

Book One

Ooh Matron!

'Ooh Matron!' is the first book in The Nomadic Nurse Series. Each book in the series takes you on a journey through medical specialisms and environments that formed part of Sarah Jane's nursing career. Throughout the series, Sarah Jane uses her trademark honest and entertaining writing style to share insights into her thoughts, reflections and the changes in her personal life and circumstances as she moves forward in her career.

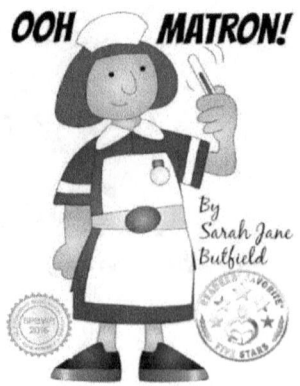

I am not sure what Florence Nightingale would have made of Sarah Jane! The story starts with a sixteen-year-old country girl who, for no apparent reason at the time, suddenly decided that she wanted to be a nurse. Sarah Jane was entering adulthood with no obvious career path in sight. She had planned a traditional, some would say old fashioned, future. Her vision was to leave school, find a job in a local store, get married and eventually have children.

Then everything changed, as she embarked on a journey which would help to map out her future by offering opportunities in a variety of places and healthcare settings. Find out how Sarah Jane deals with births, deaths and everything in between with laughter, tears and humility in this touching, sometimes heartrending, superbly written memoir.

5-star reviewers say:

"I laughed out loud at the hilarious antics, and was sobered by the genuine emotional moments that all health professionals will recognise. This is a book that will make you laugh and cry and you'll feel better for it - the perfect prescription."

"This funny, yet poignant nursing memoir has Sarah Jane's trademark honest writing style which shines through in every story she tells, from starting her student nurse training in Essex to coping with patients in happy, sad and heart-breaking situations. It gives you a young woman's view into the realities of entering the world of nursing in the 1980s. A highly entertaining and informative memoir which was able to take me from laughing out loud to having welled tears of empathy."

Available at all good bookstores on this link books2read.com/OohMatron

Bedpans to Boardrooms

Foreword	3
Introduction	8
Chapter One: At the helm of my new career as an RGN!	11
Chapter Two: Achieving a work life balance	22
Chapter Three: New beginnings	29
Chapter Four: An unusual delivery!	42
Chapter Five: Moving on up!	51
Chapter Six: New skills needed	64
Chapter Seven: Consequences and compromises	73
Chapter Eight: A new home, a new relationship and ultimately a new job!	80
Chapter Nine: All change!	87
Chapter Ten: Complex care in nursing homes	102
Chapter Eleven: Life at The Carnarvon for our residents	109
Chapter Twelve: Perception versus reality of being an aged care nurse	119
Chapter Thirteen: Upskilling and discovery!	127
Chapter Fourteen: Practicalities of independence	135
Chapter Fifteen: A new wing opens!	143
Chapter Sixteen: Let us entertain you	153
Chapter Seventeen: The Bill Versus London's Burning!	163
Chapter Eighteen: The beginning of the end	173

Sarah Jane Butfield

Epilogue Written by Shontae Brewster	183
Appendix I: Glossary of Medical Terms and Abbreviations	185
Appendix II: Reference links	186
Sneak preview of Book 3! What a mess I've made!	187
About the author, Sarah Jane Butfield	194
Keep in touch!	196
We Love Memoirs	197
Travel Memoirs by Sarah Jane Butfield	198
Other Books by Sarah Jane Butfield	205

Foreword

"Life is like a candle that burns, for the most part in a slow and steady way. However, sometimes in life, hard and challenging events occur and like gusts of wind near a candle they make the flames grow higher and the candle burns more quickly or sometimes becomes extinguished."

This analogy is taken from a conversation with one of my many, and valued, mentors that I have been fortunate to have worked alongside. This particular Matron was willing to share some of the knowledge gained during her 25 years' experience in the aged care setting. It addresses the sometimes difficult task of helping the people that you are caring for, and their relatives, deal with the acceptance of ageing and mortality in the aged care setting. For me, it helps to convey how fragile and vulnerable life is and the importance of not taking anything for granted. As my aged care career progressed, the more elderly, infirm and chronically sick people I nursed, the more relevant the words and meaning of this conversation became. It was particularly prevalent in my thoughts during the period that this book covers because it was a time, in both my personal and professional life, when I not only had to increasingly deal with death, grief and bereavement working with elderly and chronically sick adults, but also in my personal life when I experienced the death of my mother, and a second trimester miscarriage.

Aged care, nursing and residential home staff, of all grades, are often much more than simply staff members in these healthcare environments and settings. They form the backbone of an internal community that develops and exists to provide care and support, based on an ethos of respect, for the residents, their families and their individual needs. Over the years that I worked in these healthcare settings there were many challenges from both internal and external factors, such as political and regulatory change, funding and quality standard conflicts. The public perception of aged care settings during this period was sadly often a negative one. That was because it was a time when the sector became vulnerable to some unscrupulous, greedy new care home providers, before much needed regulation took the reins of quality control and patient centred care. I will share with you in this book some of my experiences and observations from a period of change in aged care. As a young, professional woman, trying to expand her professional knowledge in order to provide the best care possible, and to help and nurture staff new to this field of healthcare, I witnessed both the good, the bad and the ugly which, initially in places, appeared to be deemed acceptable when I started out as a qualified nurse. My professional responsibilities, as you will discover, changed from being focused on dispensing and administering medication, assisting with bedpans and basic personal care provision, to a time when I had an opportunity to be involved in quality led change within this sector, working in management and sitting in the boardroom of a national healthcare provider.

As I write my nursing memoirs, now fortunate to be living in picturesque South Wales, there is a quote that I see regularly on the road side when we visit Tenby, a seaside town in Pembrokeshire. It says *"The sea washes away all the ills of men."* I am not sure of its origin or history, however, it prompted me to recall numerous times, whilst working in nursing and residential homes, all situated on or near seafront locations in various Essex towns, that some residents felt soothed or more at peace by the sea. At a time when they are forced to cope with the challenges and events happening in their lives, as they pass into a new and for most final stage of acceptance in an alien environment, the sea helped to wash away their ills. I enjoy writing near the coast because my words and thoughts flow easily when I am looking out to sea and I wondered if especially the elderly found reminiscing easier in this setting.

Chronic illness and degenerative physical and mental health conditions are just a few aspects of working in the aged care sector that, at some point in our lives, we may experience either personally or through family or friends. My Beta readers say, that makes the relevance and potential appeal of this book widespread. I hope you enjoy this new

Sarah Jane Butfield

episode in my personal and professional story, including my observations, anecdotes and experiences.

Thank you for reading.

Sarah Jane Butfield

Introduction

It's the late 1980s and a newly qualified staff nurse is now taking on dual roles as she becomes a first-time mum. This additional role necessitated a rethink and some serious adjustments to her intended career pathway to enable her to juggle the roles of nurse, wife and new mum. The mortgage rates were high so the option of being a full-time stay at home mum were out of the question and in all honesty, it was not what she really wanted.

The events that follow will see Sarah Jane unexpectedly enter the aged care sector starting as a staff nurse at a private nursing and residential care facility, funded by a charitable organisation, in Colchester, Essex. Sarah Jane had trained to become a Registered General Nurse in Colchester and was familiar with the nursing home and its reputation, yet despite this familiarity with the home and her local area, this new position immediately posed challenges as she moved from the relative safety of NHS hospital wards, supported by her peers and more experienced Staff Nurses, Ward Sisters and Matrons, to a role with greater professional independence and responsibility.

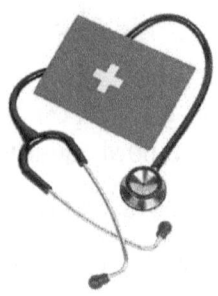

In all honesty, after completing three years of intensive study, including practical and theoretical training, passing the associated examinations and assessments, I wasn't ready to throw it all away, and that is exactly how it felt at the time! My career pathway and choices now would need to be well considered if I had any chance of utilising my nursing qualification in the future.

Work opportunities and availability were further limited by my inability to drive and the fact that at this stage Keith, my husband, was not very 'hands on' with the practical elements of our baby girl, Samantha's care. I had held a provisional driving license since the age of seventeen and had some informal driving lessons in Keith's car on the airfield at Martlesham, Suffolk, during our courting days. The need to formally learn to drive and attain my full driving licence had never risen to the top of my priority list, despite Keith buying me a car when I was 18. This now necessary skill would need to be addressed for the future if I was to cope with the multifaceted roles that I found myself trying to juggle. However, with no time, energy or money to pursue this, initially the logistics of life presented challenges that could only be dealt with by compromise and sacrifices in a variety of forms. Bearing in mind these factors it was no surprise to some of my nursing colleagues, family and friends, who had encountered similar struggles whilst trying to combine a career and a family, that I ended up working in the 'aged care' sector and outside of the NHS.

So, let's pick up where we left off in Ooh Matron and see how I went from scrubbing bedpans to sitting in the boardroom of a national nursing home group.

Chapter One: At the helm of my new career as an RGN!

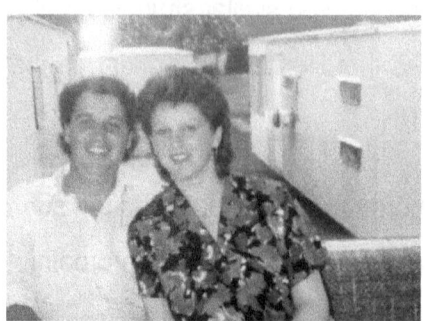

Sarah Jane and Keith

I soon settled into the role of a junior staff nurse at St Mary's Hospital. It gave me a new routine in both my work and home life, as a young married career woman. At the age of 21 with a husband of 32 it was not long after qualifying as a nurse that the question of having children arose. My new nursing career lay ahead of me now, but I also wanted a family. Of course, I had always been aware that at some stage the age difference would mean compromise by both of us. We would both want different things from our married life, at different times. Therefore, finding some common ground would take some negotiation. Whatever happened, and whenever we decided to start a family, one thing was for sure, I had to complete my six months' post registration period as an RGN, (Registered General Nurse). If not, I would have no hope of working in the NHS acute sector on my return to work. What was I even thinking about? How would I return to work after having a baby? From a financial viewpoint, there was no doubt that I would have to return to work. We had just sold our one-bedroom starter home in Wivenhoe and moved into a two-bedroom house on the same estate, as we loved it there. With no extended family living nearby to be able to help with childcare, if a return to work needed to happen, then changes at home and at work would be essential.

So how would I steer my career forwards knowing that I would need to interrupt it at some point to start a family? I had no idea. I still harboured aspirations of completing my midwifery post graduate course or pursuing a career in oncology. However, it would not be ideal to interrupt the eighteen-month course plus examinations with maternity leave. As I continued working I constantly reviewed my options. Even though the male geriatric ward was a great place to work and an ideal place to improve my skills as a junior staff nurse, I was ready for a new challenge.

In May 1987 two things happened to focus my attention on my home and work life balance. The first was that the ward sister on Ward 8, the oncology ward where I undertook my management assessment, contacted me. Before I left my oncology placement, the ward sister had said that if I was interested in a junior staff nurse position, and one became available, she would invite me to apply. If that happened it would be a huge honour and a great opportunity for any first-year staff nurse. Therefore, when the ward sister on Ward 8 called to let me know that such a position would shortly be advertised and she wondered if I would be interested my answer was, 'Hell yeah!' Well those weren't the exact words I used in that telephone conversation as you can imagine. I monitored the internal notice boards at every break time for the internal vacancy listing and the reference number needed for my application. At last it appeared and I was off, like the proverbial ferret up a drainpipe, to submit my application. This was achieved with the help of my mentor, the ward sister on the male geriatric ward. She recognised my ambitious streak and realised that I needed more than her ward could offer me. I knew that her ward was renowned for a high turnover of qualified staff, the main reason being that there was, at that time, no clear career pathway or progression within the geriatric department. With my application submitted, the waiting began. Would I be shortlisted for an interview? I was pretty confident that I would, after all I had been invited to apply. In May I received a letter informing me that I had been successful in being selected to attend an interview on Ward 8.

The second thing that happened in May was a period of sick leave from work with a stomach upset. I suspected it was due to the Chinese meal we ate the previous night after my late shift. I had been feeling nauseous all night so something I ate obviously had not agreed with me. Despite being unwell, the news that I had an interview lifted my spirits. I spent the day re-reading my oncology notes on policies, procedures, treatment regimes, etc. I wanted to be well prepared and get the job I really wanted. I would be off work for a further two days with this lingering stomach bug so I decided to take advantage of the sunny weather and read in the garden. Reading always made everything feel better.

On my return to work I was still not feeling one hundred percent. I was in the sister's office preparing the patients' notes for the doctor's ward round. With no explanation, Babs, one of the auxiliary nurses, a stocky African woman, rushed in and hugged me. She held me so tight that I felt almost unable to breathe.

"Oh, my lord, praise the lord!" She said, as she released me. "Our little Sarah has the look of motherhood about her."

"What are you talking about Babs?"

"You're glowing, beautiful girl. When are we gunna be hearing the patter of those tiny footsteps?"

"I'm not pregnant Babs, I had a stomach bug that's all."

"When was that? I didn't even know you were sick little one."

"Then why did you think I was pregnant?"

"I can see it in you. Here give me your hands?"

She took both my hands and held them tight with her eyes closed. "I see a beautiful baby girl." she said.

As she opened her eyes and released my hands I looked at her and for a split-second I wondered if she was right. Could I be pregnant? I tried to dismiss the thought as Babs put her arm around my shoulder.

"Sorry if I've upset you Sarah. I inherited this talent from my mother, just as she did from her mother."

"I'm fine Babs honestly, I'm just a bit taken aback. Don't worry when, and if, I become pregnant you will be the first to know."

Babs hugged me again and left to resume her linen trolley duties.

The rest of the day passed quickly with no more talk of babies. However, on the way to catch the bus home, my conversation with Babs replayed over and over in my head. Unintentionally the next thing I did was to walk into the chemist and bought a pregnancy testing kit. I would do the test the next morning and let Babs know that her baby radar was a bit off course on this occasion.

The presence of one blue line would indicate no pregnancy hormones in my urine. Two blue lines and I'm pregnant. As I sat in the bathroom holding the white plastic testing kit, which resembled a flattened white board marker pen, I realised that I did not have any method of timing the test. I had jumped out of bed, determined to use my first urine specimen of the day for the most accurate result, forgetting to pick up my watch from the bedside table. I didn't want to walk around holding the test, Keith did not know I would be taking a test as I didn't want him to get excited for no reason. I could hear myself counting: one Mississippi, two Mississippi, three Mississippi. We used to do that at school, playing hide and seek. I stopped when I realised how ridiculous I sounded. I looked down planning to find somewhere to place it while I went to get my watch, but there staring back at me already were two thick blue lines. Oh my god, Babs was right. But would she be right about it being a girl? I would have to wait a while to answer that one.

I didn't know what to do. Should I tell Keith now or make an appointment to see the doctor to have it confirmed before telling him? Yes, that would be the best thing to do, tell no one until the visit to the doctor. With no doctor's appointments available to fit in around my shift pattern until a week's time, I decided to put the result of the test to the back of my mind as I now faced another dilemma. Should I still attend the interview on Ward 8?

I decided that I should still go to the interview, by convincing myself that it's possible to get a false positive on a home pregnancy test. How gutted would I be if I wasn't pregnant and I passed up the opportunity of attending the interview? However, on the day of the interview, pangs of guilt invaded my thoughts. I think being in denial up until this point about the pregnancy suddenly gave way to the deep-down knowledge that I needed to accept it and face facts. I not only suffered from the morning, well actually all day, sickness and nausea, but I had this strange tingling sensation in both breasts. I also needed to pee almost hourly and on more than one occasion I wondered if I might have a urine infection instead of a positive pregnancy test. I couldn't pull out of the interview at this late stage or it would be obvious that I had known for a little while. So, I psyched myself up and headed off to Essex County Hospital. The 45-minute interview with the sister from Ward 8, and another ward sister that I didn't recognise, went better than I could ever have imagined. I managed to answer their questions with relative ease. As the interview progressed and my confidence grew, I focused so much on how well it was going and how much I wanted the job that all thoughts of a possible pregnancy completely disappeared.

I am still not quite sure how I managed to keep the news of my possible pregnancy from spilling out of my mouth, as there had been so many opportunities to say something that week, both at home and at work. Babs kept randomly hugging me, which thankfully none of the staff thought anything of, as she was a very tactile woman. Some close friends of ours announced that their first baby would be due in November, and with a guilty heart I concealed the possibility of our own baby news. Well at least for a short while longer until I was one hundred percent sure. At last the day of my doctor's appointment arrived. The treatment room nurse took my urine sample and did the equivalent of the home pregnancy test. The test involved the use of test tubes like the ones we used on the gynaecology ward during my placement there during my second year of training.

"Congratulations, you're pregnant." That's all I remember comprehending from the nurse, but I know she continued talking after that.

I was handed an appointment card for a blood test, a booklet about antenatal care services, classes and details on how to contact my local midwife. Despite having ample time to get used to the idea of being pregnant, I still walked home in a state of shock. However, by the time I reached home I was smiling with a sense of relief. The sensation of pure love for my unborn baby rushed through my body, mind and spirit. All thoughts of work and career gave way to thoughts of prams, cots and an overwhelming desire to tell the world!

Keith, as expected, was over the moon when I told him the news, as were both of our families. At work, I didn't know when to announce it, but for the health and safety of myself, our baby and my colleagues it needed to be soon. At that time, we still manually lifted patients and frequently used 'The Australian Lift'. This was a two-nurse manoeuvre that involved putting your shoulder under the patient's armpit while facing the top of the bed. Then clasping wrists under the patient's thighs with your partner before lifting them up the bed. This put a huge strain on your neck and back muscles. The crouched position would become increasingly uncomfortable as my pregnancy developed and there was no way I was going to risk losing my baby. So, at the earliest opportunity I told the ward sister who immediately relieved me of all lifting duties.

Babs, the one person I wanted to share my news with, was on annual leave. I didn't like that everyone else on the ward was finding out about the baby before her as I had promised she would be the first to know. I need not have worried. Babs returned to work with a 'Congratulations' card and a beautiful pot plant called a Cyclamen. With my pregnancy hormones in full flow my tears of happiness fell frequently.

A week later the letter, which previously I would have anxiously awaited, but now had almost completely forgotten about, arrived. It informed me that my application had been successful for the position of junior staff nurse on Ward 8 at Essex County Hospital. Now the reality of deciding how I would manage my career and a family started to kick in. I would need to return to work, if only for financial reasons. We had a mortgage that could not be covered by one income, especially with a family to support. These events all occurred during the 1980s property boom, but, would I be able to work and manage hospital shifts with a new baby? Who would care for my baby? The more I thought about it the more confused and unsure I became. I felt selfish at the thought of accepting a role that I would need to leave in a few months' time, especially as the ward sister had been encouraging enough to invite me to apply. I made a conscious decision that I would not let worrying about what might happen after my baby was born spoil my pregnancy and I declined the position, albeit with a heavy heart. I took the very blinkered view of, 'We will deal with that when and if the time comes,' ever hopeful that something might change to make the decision easier.

After a period of sick leave for hypertension (raised blood pressure) I started my maternity leave and Samantha Louise was born in December 1987. She was born three weeks early in an induced labour after I developed pre-eclampsia, a complication of pregnancy which demonstrated itself with symptoms including hypertension, swelling (oedema) and protein (proteinuria) in my urine due to the extra strain on my kidneys.

Not long after the birth the decision I had deferred needed to be addressed. I had to work out how and when I would be able to make a financial contribution to our household income. The only skill that would earn me the maximum amount of money for the least number of hours worked was nursing. All my maternal instincts told me to stay at home with my new baby, but the need for me to return to work in the months that followed did not abate. Even so, I did not initially contemplate returning to work full-time. So, when I did return it was not to my staff nurse position at St Mary's in the NHS, instead I would now have my first experience of working for a non-profit organisation providing aged care services in nursing and residential homes around Colchester. I became a part time (weekend) staff nurse at Cheviot Nursing Home.

The Balkerne Garden Trust charity owned Cheviot Residential and Nursing Care facility in Colchester, near to where I trained as a nurse. However, it was a world away from the work and the environment I was familiar with. Gone was the safe, secure and supported setting of an acute hospital working alongside my peers and an array of senior staff from a multitude of specialities. Now I found myself working weekends and night shifts with much less support, necessary so that I could work when Keith was at home to care for Samantha. I would often be part of a small workforce and later found myself in charge with the only help, advice or guidance being available at the end of the telephone from the senior RGN on call.

I quickly realised that this was 'normal' in aged care and I was told on one occasion, when I dared to voice my concerns about the apparent lack of hands on support for the qualified nurses that, "I was lucky to be working in a charity run organisation, and that staffing levels and working conditions were often lower, and conditions much worse, in the privately owned homes whose primary focus was on profit, closely followed by the resident's care, with the needs of the staff taking a very low priority." Over the years that followed I would learn first-hand that this was true.

New developments in my career waited in the wings, preparing to open, but at this time little did I know what lay ahead and what compromises and sacrifices, both personal and professional, I would have to make.

Chapter Two: Achieving a work life balance

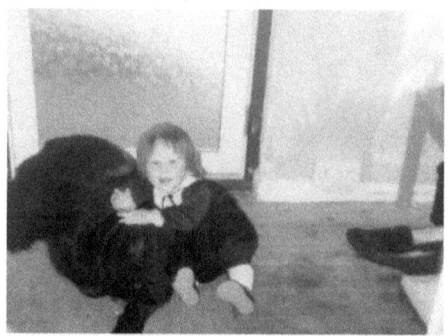

Samantha with our dog Sophie during our house renovations

As Keith and I entered 1988 as a working couple with a baby and now a new Collie cross dog called Sophie, we fitted or resembled the stereotypical perfect small family unit and from the outside our life probably looked idyllic and relatively easy. We visited our extended family when we had time off together on weekends or during holidays. Our house, albeit with a mortgage bigger than we planned due to the 1980s-housing boom, was positioned in a riverside village where we had developed a nice circle of friends locally, as our larger circle of friends were back in Suffolk where we originated from. I had, by necessity, returned to work very early after Samantha was born. I didn't qualify for the full period of maternity pay from the NHS as my period of service hadn't started until I took up my role as an RGN, when I qualified. After a few weeks emergency financial action was required.

Despite the mortgage rates being high we had, before I found out that I was pregnant with Samantha, moved out of our one bedroom starter home and into to a two-bedroom town house on the same estate in Wivenhoe. The addition of an extra bedroom, a small garden and allocated parking, which pleased Keith who was a bit of a petrol head, appeared to be worth the investment. However, after Samantha was born we quickly realised that the additional bedroom we had acquired was no match for the equipment needed with a new baby in the house. In reality, it was a box room that most people would use for the storage of the ironing board and suitcases!

As we reviewed our options both financially and practically, we decided that the only course of action was to move to a cheaper area where we could get more house for the same money. We could not afford to pay more, if anything, we needed to pay less. As Wivenhoe is situated in a picturesque waterfront location we knew that we would have no problem selling and for a good price, so we started our house hunt in earnest heading along the Essex coastline. We had to be conscious of Keith's travel to work, but at that time he was working for a piling company in London and his commute was already extensive. Therefore, we took on the more challenging task of not only finding a new home, but also that of trying to find Keith a new job.

Our hope, and ideal scenario, would be that if Keith had a shorter commute it would give him more quality family time at home and facilitate me returning to work as a nurse. That way, I could earn a higher hourly rate than he could as an unskilled, although hard working, labourer. I already had work as a part-time staff nurse, working weekends and nights, which involved a small amount of travel, therefore I was acutely aware that the further we moved the less viable it would be for me to work in Colchester. Public transport on weekends was notoriously poor at that time for shift workers. The further we moved away, the less feasible it would be for Keith to drive me to work then come back six or eight hours later. Samantha was obviously uppermost in our thoughts during these considerations, since she would be in bed asleep during some of these journeys. Our daily conversations and thoughts were consumed with coming up with options, ideas and potential actions, until finally we found the ideal house for the same money we currently paid. It was a large, semi-detached, ex-council house on a corner plot with a big fenced garden. To Keith's delight it also had three, brick built outbuildings and a driveway suitable for two cars which meant he could work on his motoring projects and leave his tools and oily rags wherever he wanted. It also gave him the space to store his prized sea fishing equipment which had always been a challenge in the previous houses, when it ended up being stored at his mother's house in Debenham, Suffolk. This dictated that, without a lot of extra travelling time, he could only go fishing when we visited Suffolk, which became less frequent the more I needed to work on weekends and thus limited access to the hobby which he loved.

Although aged care had not been the area of nursing I anticipated working in when I qualified, after a few months at Cheviot I began to wonder if it was indeed my vocation. I really enjoyed the interaction with the residents, even though I did miss the buzz of acute care nursing. I loved listening to their stories while I attended to their medication needs, dressings or personal care. Some of the very personal stories that have been told and that were entrusted to me during my career still make my heart tingle when I reflect on them today. There is so much knowledge, experience, and humility hidden in the hearts and minds of elderly and infirm people. Far too often there is no opportunity or desire for anyone to listen to them. For many elderly people a move to an aged care facility means the loss of their home, their possessions, all bar possibly a favourite chair, some ornaments or a bedspread, although probably nowadays this is less often achieved due to health and safety regulations. However, at Cheviot the residents were encouraged to have familiar items brought in to give their new room a sense of home and to induce calm and tranquillity. I loved looking at the photographs many of them would have adorning the walls. Often, they were of their wedding day or their family members, when their children were babies or toddlers. Others would have pictures of their children and grandchildren at special life changing times such as weddings, births, joining the armed forces, university graduations, etc.

To ensure that I gained the most from my part time working hours, to continue my professional development as a newly qualified nurse, I pushed myself forward for places on study days and courses as they became available. Again, I soon realised that I was fortunate to be working in a well-funded charity organisation which made investing money in their staff a priority and not an after-thought like some private homes that I would later experience. Unlike the NHS, funds for training were available for candidates who submitted a comprehensive application on how the training or study would impact the provision of nursing care, and the performance of their role, after the course. I enjoyed learning developing the ability to write a compelling case for why I should be chosen, another skill that would serve me well later.

At this time, nursing as a profession, both in the NHS and private sector, was undergoing change. Some areas of compliance and regulation, that had previously been ruled and monitored with recommendations for best practice, were moving towards these being requirements that would be rigorously enforced and increasingly regulated, to improve standards of both patient /resident care and staff training across the board. These changes focused on accountability, and improving care planning practice and implementation by starting to use a formal, documented holistic approach, where the input came not only from the qualified nurses' professional medical assessment of the residents needs. It also involved the valuable input from the care assistants who contributed more on the physical limitations and capabilities of the individuals concerned. Further improvements over the years were leading towards a time when care assistants, or as they are now known, health care assistants, move ever closer to being licensed, regulated and protected in the same way that nurses are.

In past times it was common-place for care assistants to be trained in-house by their peers and sometimes the qualified nurses, if time and resources permitted, working 'on the job'. Because of this, some new care assistants who arrived with little or no prior experience often acquired bad habits if they were unlucky enough to be inducted by an existing care assistant with questionable standards. It was from the acknowledgement of this problem that internal improvement practices and quality assurance programs, both locally and nationally, started to focus on the need for some form of accreditation for care assistants. Fortunately for the residents, nurses, care and ancillary staff, where I worked, the executive committee, that managed the charity, were very proactive at pushing this measure through and funding the education of the staff they employed. It became a huge retention factor and as such you can probably imagine my severe reservations at even the consideration of leaving to find work nearer to our new home in healthcare environments who would possibly now struggle to meet my newly acquired raised expectations of support and quality led standards of care in the aged care sector.

In hindsight, although I could not play a major part in the implementation of quality systems, policies and procedures due to my part time hours and my junior status, I did develop a deep-seated interest in quality and compliance and how this is best achieved by quality led training and resources provided by passionate individuals who believe in adding value to the resident's experiences by investing in the staff around them. The prospect of leaving this inspirational and proactive workplace to do who knows what or where was not appealing, but the reality was that as I couldn't drive and I had to put my family and our financial requirements first, the sacrifice for now would be to my career. Never did I expected that compromise to be as large or influential as it turned out to be.

Chapter Three: New beginnings

Our new home was in the small coastal town of Brightlingsea, Essex. Brightlingsea is situated midpoint between Colchester and Clacton at the mouth of the River Colne. Although historically a fishing and shipbuilding town it has long since lost all connections with industry. Since the loss of the railway link to nearby Wivenhoe in the 1960s it had become a boat lovers' tourist attraction and a popular seaside resort for young families due to its beach huts, lack of expensive fun fair rides and amusement arcades and the presence of a shallow water pool at the beach front, although the water quality and colour of the children as they emerged from it left a lot to be desired.

In the 1980s and 90s, with property prices soaring, its location offered affordable housing to families with their own transport whilst still providing the opportunity to shop, bank and access leisure facilities in neighbouring towns or the ability to shop locally with a supermarket, post office, banks and other small shops in the High Street. The town centre was an easy walk for me with a pushchair and we found that once a week or fortnight was frequent enough to go the larger supermarkets in Colchester. The other advantage of our new location for Keith was the proximity to the sea now that he had his precious sea fishing gear safely stowed away in this array of outbuildings. He also acquired a small boat one night in the pub. I think he won it in a game of dice, which was usual for him. Ever since we first met he had a knack for winning random items at the bar of his local pub. He would come home with joints of meat, dead animals which he assured me we could eat and items of interest to a motor junkies like himself - bits of old vehicles or even a whole wrecked car once. He liked to play dice, darts and most pub games and although not a gambler he would wager items over money, but that's another story!

I started my nursing job search in earnest, but quickly became disheartened as I realised that my options were either to continue to work in Colchester with the inconvenience and upheaval it imposed on Samantha, or to work locally, but not as a nurse.

With no NHS hospital in Brightlingsea, and only a small GP practice which was not an area of nursing that I had any experience in, I turned to the local residential homes. Initially I was surprised at the number of offers I received, until I realised that the acquisition of a qualified nurse being prepared to work and be paid as a care assistant made the private home owners rub their hands together. The prospect for them was of offloading some responsibility, and raising the standards in their establishment, without upfront investment. Residential homes, at that time, did not require a qualified nurse team, although most were operated by retired RGN's who had the experience to set them up and the managerial skills to ensure a degree of compliance. However, as time went on more homes were opening in seemingly ordinary houses, especially in Clacton where large, seafront Victorian houses became well suited to offering prestigious sea views with residential and nursing care for exorbitant fees. In Brightlingsea it was residential and care homes only and because the pay rates were so much less than I had been earning either as a student nurse or as a junior staff nurse in aged care, I had no choice but to take on two jobs to ensure that I had enough shifts to make the money we needed.

The first place I started work at was called Oakland's, a smaller home for 14 residents at that time and not far from the town centre. It was easily accessible for me by bicycle and it was run by an Asian family, who had very high expectations of their staff and tried to deliver a cost-effective service to their residents. They were one of the few homes at the time who took their residents out on excursions and shopping trips, which was one of their unique selling points, but for staff like me, particularly on nights, the regimes were hard work physically, although not mentally taxing. I do not know if in the past, they had been subject to criticism of their cleanliness, but they had some borderline obsessive cleaning regimes in place. The worst of these for me was the nightly hand scrubbing of the kitchen floor with Ajax powder, after I had done the vegetable preparation for the following day. For those of you not familiar with Ajax powder it is a hard-abrasive powdered household and industrial cleaning product. It had a strong odour and contained blue crystal like particles. Its distinctive smell, and the way it harshly roughened the skin on my hands if I didn't wear gloves is something I will never forget. Aside from this, the personal care needed by the residents was well within my skill set and I enjoyed it. The medication was administered by the owners before they left each evening. I worked two nights a week here.

My second place of employment was Well House Residential Home which was owned by the local council and was home to 48 residents who were divided up into four smaller units - one was residential and low dependency, one was EMI (Elderly, Mental, Infirm) high dependency and the other two were medium dependency. There were a mixture of male and female residents and the care needs ranged from supervision of self caring activities, to total care of all aspects of daily living, for example mobility, feeding, hygiene and so on.

Even though Well House was classified as a residential home for registration purposes, in my professional opinion the level of expertise needed for individual resident's needs, especially in the high dependency unit, bordered on a nursing care skillset. In addition to personal care and observation duties once a week the night staff had the unappealing task of scrubbing the metal bedpans and deep cleaning the sinks in the sluices. I think it must have been the way my shift pattern fell that dictated that I appeared to always be on duty when this had to be done. Either that or the other staff made it work that way! There was another night staff duty which always reminded me of Paddington Bear, this involved making three large platters of white bread and marmalade sandwiches for the residents' breakfasts the next morning, although we would sometimes make some of the early risers a couple of slices of toast as a treat!

The early risers were not always up through personal choice. There were a couple of the long-standing night shift care assistants who, supposedly because of the 'low daytime staffing levels', operated a practice of early get ups, which was controversial at the time, and I believe still is. The residents in the high dependency unit, who were in the main mentally impaired, would be woken usually around 4.30am, washed, dressed and sat in the lounge, to give the day staff a 'head start' on getting everybody up and ready for breakfast by 8am. Given that most of the residents in this wing were incontinent, the process of getting them up washed and dressed at the tail end of a 12-hour night shift was a tough ask. For me, personally and physically, this practice would soon become much more difficult. I think the local authorities had received tip offs about this practice because some of the care assistants seemed overly prepared for questions that they might be asked about why they were washing and dressing residents at this early hour if an unannounced spot check visit occurred. Their answers included, 'The resident was incontinent and needed a full bed bath and it wasn't worth putting them back into pyjamas.'

I was acutely aware that working as a care assistant whilst holding an RGN qualification would leave me in a vulnerable position from a professional indemnity, liability and accountability perspective. As a registered nurse, I had the nursing code of conduct and a duty of care to abide by in whatever position I worked. I had to be very careful not to let myself be placed into situations where I would be utilising my professional qualification and skills in a non-qualified, paid position. This turned out to be a tricky balancing act, requiring tact and diplomacy, when dealing with the residential home owners and management, to avoid confrontation. Especially so with those who were themselves unqualified in general nursing. I think it is a natural reaction, when you know how to do something, to want to step straight in and do it or assist. However, the perceived 'nursing or responsible person' tasks were the sole responsibility of the home owners or managers and although they did sometimes try to delegate them to me I had to resist the urge to agree to help. I was aware of, and had discussed these scenarios with a Royal College of Nursing union representative previously before I undertook my first care assistant role at St Mary's Hospital whilst waiting for my nurse registration documents to come through. I felt confused and torn between my personal and professional accountabilities and responsibilities. I therefore knew what the potential pitfalls were of blurring the lines between the roles of a care assistant and a nurse.

Residential homes, with no access to on-site qualified nursing staff, relied on the local GP surgery, (General Practice doctors), out of hours' services and the district nursing team for insulin injections, wound care, dealing with asthma attacks, etc. and even though these too were well within my experience and skill set, I had to refrain from any involvement in dealing with these activities despite a lot of pressure. The misuse of the out of hours' services, sometimes blatantly wasting a GP's time and calling them out for events that could wait for a routine appointment, did not help with the already bad reputation that some residential homes in the area had acquired. However, the home owners were quick to gloat when a nearby home or owner was pulled to task over this, even though many of them were also guilty of these practices.

As there were no regulatory requirements, at that time, for the formal training or ongoing skills assessment of care assistants, the standard of care provision in some homes was shocking and inadequate. As members of the care staff in residential homes with a good local reputation we often only heard the horror stories of bad practices from new care staff being employed or residents who left the poorly managed homes. Some of the horror stories even made the local press due to families reporting the home and their owners to the local authorities, which at that time supported the funding of some residential care home placements on a means tested basis. The other side effect of bad practice in other local homes was that unfortunately some care assistants had their first experience of working in aged care in these poorly run homes and they believed the care they had been trained in-house to give was of a good standard. Consequently, when we tried to coach and retrain them some resistance was met, particularly by the older care assistants who resented a younger persons input. I think I was perceived by some as having a 'stuck up' personality attributed to the fact that I was a qualified nurse. Some of them took every opportunity to belittle me and the way I preferred to deliver basic personal care to our residents, but I would not compromise just to be liked by them.

These factors prayed on my mind during this period of my career. I use the word 'career' with a degree of sadness because I truly felt that I had let my career drift away from me and that there was little hope of getting it back on track any time soon. I was acutely aware that I could not afford, from a professional viewpoint, to be involved in any sub-standard work practices or be employed in homes that condoned them as I had my professional reputation to consider. Having worked as a care assistant, and as a nurse, I could see both sides of the many arguments that were debated. I quickly became aware of how undervalued, and unappreciated, care assistants were made to feel. This was the reason why many homes had constant staffing problems as care staff would not stay to be treated in that way when new homes were opening, or being expanded, throughout Essex as month by month, more funding became available.

The registration of residential care homes during this period came under the remit of a special division of Essex County Council and in their efforts to improve standards and enhance the public perception of this industry, which was expanding, they did implement a range of planned and unplanned on-site inspections. In very basic terms if a residential home failed an inspection they were given notice to resolve the issues. If they consistently failed to do this or were found to slip back into bad practice procedures later, they could be removed from the approved provider listing which would mean that the only residents they would be able to accommodate would be those who were fully privately funded with no social services or local authority top up. During this period that represented a small proportion of the residents looking for care and so avoiding this penalty was a high priority.

At Oaklands the routine for working nights as a care assistant was different. It consisted of getting residents settled into bed for the night, answering their call bells when they needed the toilet or a change of position and preparing the vegetables for the following day's meals. When this was done the night time cleaning commenced. I enjoyed the practical care elements, but meal preparation and cleaning were not tasks that I enjoyed at home and I liked them even less whilst trying to complete them during the night when I was already tired from being a mum during the day, with limited sleep. The owners were an Asian family and they would leave out an array of vegetables for me to prepare. Some, at that time, I was unfamiliar with and I didn't know how to prepare them. Should I peel them, scrub them, chop, dice or slice them? At night, I was the only member of staff awake, the other care assistant was on what was called 'a sleep over shift' and I was only to wake her in an emergency as she would be working as the day time care assistant the whole of the next day. This meant that if I woke her for something that the owners felt was not an emergency then there were stern words of reprimand that would be spoken. This was because if she was woken, she was entitled to be paid as an awake care assistant for the whole night and could only work half of the following day shift. This then required staff cover to be sourced at short notice the next day. Any actions that were deemed unwarranted and increased the wages bill were unpopular to say the least. The owners soon recognised my vegetable identification and preparation ignorance and they started leaving examples of what they wanted done with them in the kitchen. On one occasion, they even left me a picture cut out of a magazine. The cleaning tasks were extreme in both depth and technique, but not in sophistication. The lino flooring in the kitchen was scrubbed with Ajax and a nail brush each night after the vegetable and meal preparation was complete. This was then followed by cold water mopping before buffing it dry with a large towel.

It was during one of these nightly cleaning regimes that I experienced an event that would change things for me and my career again. I was bent over on my hands and knees on the kitchen floor as usual when I felt something strange in my abdomen. Initially, it resembled the flutter of nervousness just before an interview, but then it took on a stronger, more physical sensation which I can only describe as prodding. It was not a pain it was more like I was being prodded with something, but from the inside. My female brain, having experienced the kicks of pregnancy before, identified with the sensation, but I quickly dismissed it as impossible as I had a coil in situ for contraception and I was still expressing breast milk for Samantha.

This dismissal caused me to engage an over-reacting nursing assessment of my symptoms. What life threatening condition could cause this sensation? I sat upright on the floor, leaning my back against the kitchen unit doors, and placed my hand on my abdomen. Was I going to die? Maybe I had an aortic aneurysm? I was getting myself worked up trying to figure out what I should do as I was technically alone caring for the residents. Should I wake the sleep-in carer? I decided that I needed to calm myself down. I didn't feel ill, so maybe it was wind! I stood myself up and started to make a cup of tea. As I waited for the kettle to boil the fluttering settled and I convinced myself that I had totally over reacted and I was relieved that I hadn't woken the carer. On my way home the next morning whilst riding my bicycle the fluttering sensation started again. I decided that I would walk to the doctors after Keith left for work and I had fed and dressed Samantha, to book an appointment to check this out.

I walked into the doctor's surgery and Patricia the receptionist said that, if I wanted to wait, she had an appointment in 30 minutes. I was tired from my night shift and all I wanted was to get home and lay down, but my apprehension over my condition persuaded me to accept her offer. I sat down and before long I could feel my head nodding as my body craved sleep.

This dozing sensation was shattered when Patricia said, "Sarah, you can go in now. Do you want me to watch Samantha for you?"

"Ok, oh, yes thank you."

In the consulting room, I explained my fluttering and prodding experiences as the doctor checked my blood pressure, listened to my heart and palpated my abdomen. The doctor asked me to give a urine specimen to the nurse and wait in the reception area until it was tested, then she would see me again. I did as I was instructed and I was soon called back in again.

"Congratulations, Sarah it seems you are pregnant. As you are experiencing movements I think we should get an ultra sound scan carried out as soon as possible. You could be at least 16 weeks pregnant. Let me make a call to see if we can get you an appointment today."

"That's impossible, I have a coil!"

"It can happen, but you don't need to worry, the likelihood of the baby being affected when you have reached this stage of pregnancy is unlikely, but we do need to take a look and see how things are progressing."

"It must be a mistake, what else could cause this?"

"Let's get the scan done and take it from there, ok?"

I had no choice than to call Keith as the scan appointment was for that afternoon. As we sat in the radiology department that afternoon I was still convinced that I would not be seeing a baby on the screen. When they rolled the scanning probe across my abdomen, muttering as they took measurements, I thought I was going to pass out when she said, "It looks like you're 20 weeks and 2 days. You have missed your early blood tests and with the baby being at 20 weeks gestation we need to be testing for Downs Syndrome. We will send you over to pathology to get those tests done now."

Shock and disbelief flooded my thoughts, I looked at Keith who really didn't seem to understand the impact of what we had just been told. He was just excited that we were expecting another child as he really wanted a boy at some stage.

After a walk to the pathology laboratory, I had my blood test and was given instructions to make an appointment with my doctor in three days to get the results and to be booked in for antenatal services. By the time we arrived home I realised that I had neither eaten or slept since finishing work at 7am that morning, so Keith took care of Samantha and I had a nap on the sofa. Keith ordered a Chinese takeaway for dinner. Luckily, I was not due to work that night so I had time to try and come to terms with the day's revelations.

The news of our new baby, which would be due in late September, was well received by our family and friends and for a few weeks I tried not to think of the practicalities of how we would manage with two babies under two years old both from a financial and logistical point of view.

Chapter Four: An unusual delivery!

I am not entirely sure if it was the conflict I still felt working as a care assistant whilst holding a nursing qualification or if it was my raging pregnancy hormones, but for the following few weeks I struggled with mood swings, extreme fatigue and random emotional outbursts at work. Little did I know at the time that I was in the verge of developing pre-eclampsia, but I did know that whatever happened I needed to remove the professional dilemma from my life sooner rather than later. Although I had consciously decided to resolve this, even considering and applying for jobs as a cleaner in non-healthcare environments to completely remove the professional risk, Mother Nature intervened at 33 weeks, taking the decision out of my hands. My blood pressure soared as pre-eclampsia took hold and I was immediately admitted to hospital for rest in the hope that not working and not having to care for an active toddler would settle my condition. It didn't, but what I experienced led to deep rooted memories which have stayed with me ever since.

As I had previously worked as a student nurse at the maternity hospital I knew most of the qualified midwives on the antenatal ward and because of this I was admitted to a side room. My rose-tinted view of the perceived 'nice gesture' of giving me a side room was soon changed. I remember as a student thinking how nice it must be for patients to get a side room, but at a time of extreme anxiety for my unborn baby and for my own health, as I knew the potential issues of pre-eclampsia, I craved the company and camaraderie of other expectant mums and the reassurance of the midwifery staff going about their duties. It turns out that the real reason for the side room was to prevent me from possibly filling the other prospective mums heads with labour horror stories! Everyone knows that nurses make the worst patients and stories from inside the NHS had a habit of leaking out.

I discovered from Carol, a friendly enrolled nurse, that there had been instances of staff as patients demanding special treatment and when they didn't get it they had criticised the maternity unit to other patients. Once, a story even made its way into the local newspaper. If you can imagine being a first-time mother, with raging pregnancy hormones, filled with anxiety and feeling unwell hearing nurses talking badly about the unit or its staff, then the use of the side room was probably a good, preventative measure.

My blood pressure showed no signs of reducing and the other symptoms of pre-eclampsia escalated, with severely swollen legs and fingers, pounding headaches and disturbed vision plaguing my body. I struggled to get any meaningful periods of rest as my fatigue increased. Reluctantly after a week in hospital suffering from sleep deprivation I gave in and agreed to take some mild night sedation. I was prescribed Temazepam 10 - 20mgs to try to induce sleep to my exhausted body and growing baby. The first couple of nights I took the 10mg dose and it produced little in the way of solid sleep so, on the 23rd August, I reluctantly agreed to take a 20mg dose. In hindsight, I wonder if I am just a control freak, (yes, I know you can't believe that of me,) and maybe I had fought the effects of the sedation on the previous nights, because it took only minutes for the higher dose to kick in as I tried to read my 'Mother and Baby' magazine.

I awoke with a warm, damp sensation under my bottom and lower back. Thinking that I had wet the bed due to my deep, drug induced sleep, I knew that I needed to get up and deal with this situation. I looked at the white-faced clock on the wall in front of me and saw that it was only 2.20 am. As I moved, intending to head off to the bathroom to sort out my embarrassing accident, I suddenly felt a pressure on my inner thigh. I threw back the sheets, looked and screamed. Carol, an already loud, American nurse ran in and also started screaming.

Suddenly from behind her came the ward sisters loud, assertive instruction. "Keep still Sarah!"

As Carol grabbed a wheelchair she shouted, "Donna, call the delivery suite and tell them we are on the way. Tell them to page the on-call anaesthetist and his team."

Carol pulled the wheelchair close to edge of the bed. I was crying, fearing the worst for my baby, whose head I could now feel properly between my legs.

"Now let's get you to the labour ward," Carol spluttered, obviously still trying to regain her own composure after her initial outburst, as she gently manoeuvred my legs to the side of the bed.

"Is the baby ok?"

"Everything is just swell, now come on with you."

"I can't sit in that chair!" I shouted.

"Yes, you can, I will position you, don't worry." Worry was not the word I would have used to describe my feelings at that moment. Hysteria would probably be more appropriate. As Carol and the ward sister pulled me to a standing position a student midwife, who had been watching this debacle from the doorway, suddenly lurched forwards. I don't know exactly what happened in that split second, but I felt a tugging sensation as she grabbed the bed sheet and it disappeared from its role of covering my dignity. The next thing I knew she was sprawled beneath me. I felt as if my intestines had dropped from my body as a large squelch echoed and Carol screamed again.

The screaming was immediately replaced with a shout of, "I've got it!" from the student midwife.

"Bloody hell!" Donna shouted, as she rushed back from making the telephone calls, "You've had your baby, Sarah."

I felt faint, my legs wobbled and a hot sweat came over me. They pushed me backwards onto the bed and I think I must have passed out for a minute or two because as my eyes opened, despite the room spinning I could hear Carol saying, "That's it, placenta is out and intact." I was shaking uncontrollably as they cut the cord and started rolling me from side to side to change the blood and amniotic fluid soaked bedding.

The next half an hour found me in an undignified position which involved me laying with my legs up in stirrups. The ward sister and the student midwife inspected and sutured various parts of my perineum which had been torn in the process of my baby making its unannounced, sudden, premature entry into the world with no labour pains or preparation.

Turning towards Carol I hardly dared to ask, "Is it alive?"

No answer.

I wondered if they had they called Keith. I could feel tears running down my face as I lay out of control of my body, my baby and my emotions. Too much silence prevailed to reassure me until a nurse, in a bright pink tabard, from the Special Care Baby Unit (SCBU) appeared holding a Polaroid picture of my baby. She handed me the picture and started talking me through what I was looking at.

"You have a beautiful baby boy, he is a little jaundiced and his oxygen levels are a little unstable so he is in the ventilator as a precaution. We struggled to get some IV (Intravenous) access into his tiny veins and so we had to access a vein via his scalp." I studied the picture again and I could see his partially shaved scalp with an intravenous line in place.

"Will he be ok? I want to go and see him now." I tried to pull myself out of the stirrups and up to a sitting position, but a humming noise filled my head and the room was spinning again.

"Let the midwife finish getting you sorted out, they will get you some tea and toast and by that time the doctors will have completed their checks. Then we will have all the answers you need," the SCBU nurse said, trying to reassure me.

I didn't think I needed tea or toast until I tried to stand to transfer to the wheelchair and realised how weak I was both from the trauma of the delivery and the after effects of the night sedation. Sitting in the wheelchair I felt like a sleepy pensioner on the bus with my head nodding, backwards and forwards. Then a voice stirred my consciousness again.

"Welcome back Sarah!"

I had passed out again. I now had a drip in my left arm and as the fluids entered my veins I immediately started to feel better. Once they were sure I was ready to try again the staff helped me into my clean maternity nightdress and I was soon being wheeled to SCBU.

As we travelled through the corridors the student midwife asked, "Didn't you feel any of the contractions?" She was obviously curious to know more about how this birth escalated so fast without me calling for help.

As my thoughts trawled back over the events of the last couple of hours, so that I could answer her, I realised that I hadn't thanked her for the rugby tackle style dive she made to stop my baby boy landing on the floor.

"I can never thank you enough for your quick thinking and actions, you saved him!"

"To be honest I don't remember thinking, I just saw what was happening and threw myself at your feet, it's a bit surreal to be honest."

In SCBU the cots were lined up against the wall with monitors, oxygen tubes, suction apparatus and IV stands surrounding them in an orderly fashion. I was parked in my wheelchair beside my baby boy who was encased in his ventilated cot.

"Can I hold him?"

"We will pop some nasal cannulas in to keep him on the oxygen therapy then you can hold him and try him on the breast." She continued to explain about the importance of skin to skin contact for SCBU babies, but I wasn't listening I just wanted to hold him. When he was finally cradled in my arms the tears started flowing again as did the colostrum from my nipples.

I studied every inch of my baby boy from his head, complete with intravenous drip, to his chest with three tiny electrodes that traced his heartbeats, down to his ten tiny toes.

Keith arrived in a fluster, but there was no disguising his joy when he found out that he had a son, because as much as he loved Samantha, he longed for a son who would grow up to share his love of cars, fishing and outdoor pursuits. As it turned out it was Samantha, our little 'tom boy', who participated in more of these things than her brother.

I know all mums spend what feels like their whole lives in the early days wanting their babies to stop crying, but right now all I wanted to hear was my little boy cry. He did eventually, and he would make up for his subdued start in the weeks and months that followed. Back on the post-natal ward just when I needed the seclusion of a side room there were now none available and I joined the other mums, most of whom had babies in cots beside them. I felt empty and a failure, as I berated myself for choosing sleeping tablets over the health of my baby. I know it wasn't really like that but, as my pregnancy hormones rampaged through me combined with exhaustion, that was the simplistic rationale that I created for myself.

We named our baby boy Robert Andrew Parker.

Chapter Five: Moving on up!

Despite the pregnancy ending in a traumatic fashion, resulting in Robert staying in SCBU, I still had my other baby Samantha at home to think about and Keith needed to return to work, as there was no paid paternity leave available in those days. I ended up at home expressing breast milk on a pumping machine, lent to me by the SCBU unit. It was heavy, noisy and painful to use and made me feel sorry for cows at milking time. But it was necessary to enable me to give Robert the best start in life and it meant I could take bottles of breast milk to the SCBU nursery every day for him.

In a few weeks, he was home, but because of my delayed start to being a stay at home mum of two, all too quickly the honeymoon, or 'babymoon,' period was over and the phrase I now dreaded reared its ugly head – returning to work! It became the main topic of conversation, debate and worry. How was I going to combine being a new mum with two babies under two years of age with shift work that fitted in around Keith's work? Even though I had known during my pregnancy that I would have to return to work quickly, the reality of it was very hard to accept. It put a strain on our marriage as we became consumed with just coping instead of living and enjoying our little family. Keith was doing everything he could to earn, or make, extra money and he was still working on the renovations in our home to make the babies' room more suitable to accommodate our new addition.

The answer was that I had to return to work as a care assistant in the residential home, but this time I had to work one night on and one night off as I had no opportunity to sleep during the day to be able to work consecutive nights. The process of reminiscing, recalling and writing about it now brings back the sense of constant tiredness that I felt operating this arduous, sleep deprived routine. After my night shift, which was always physically exhausting, I would try to settle Robert in his pram and put Samantha in her playpen so that I could lay on the sofa and doze whilst trying to stay alert enough to hear them if they needed anything. In reality I was so afraid of not hearing them that I couldn't even doze off.

It quickly became obvious that this arrangement was not going to work in the long term. I needed the same money, but for working less hours and the only way to achieve that was to return to work as an RGN. Now came the how and where? As I already knew there were no RGN opportunities in Brightlingsea my search area had to be expanded to Colchester and Clacton. I initially tried to search using the availability of public transport to help me define the jobs I could apply for. I looked for the hours I could potentially work, in roles within my skill set and most importantly ensuring that Keith or close friends could be available to help with childcare.

This scenario presented too many obstacles and I had to go back to the drawing board. Plan B meant working out Keith's ability to take me to work and collect me with minimal disruption to our babies. I knew the degree of flexibility that I needed in relation to my working hours could only come from one sector; aged care. Clacton was a boom town for new nursing homes from the late 1980s. Property investors had recognised the potential of large seafront Victorian buildings that could easily be converted into single and double rooms, which would command very profitable weekly fees for both private and social services funded placements. My aged care experience as a junior staff nurse and then as a care assistant, up until this point, in hindsight, revealed how naïve I was to the way home owners and nursing home companies would recruit, use and treat qualified nurses. I had a huge learning curve ahead of me.

I was pleasantly surprised at how easy it was to find positions to apply for, despite regarding myself as inexperienced in this field. I was interviewed and offered a position on my first outing, which gave me a huge professional boost. I subsequently discovered that it was not hard for anyone with a qualification to find the exact hours they wanted. The increase in the number of homes opening, and the staffing requirements they had, meant that there was always a deficit of qualified nursing staff. Seaside towns across the country were seeing these trends, and as the demand grew the acquisition of large, potentially suitable buildings spread inland. Developers obviously preferred buildings that had previously been hotels or guest houses as these had a large proportion of the conversion work already completed meaning they could get their aged care rooms to market quicker. The challenge then for this growing sector was finding and retaining quality staff because, staff very quickly recognised their potential value and would move and negotiate their own terms with homes desperate for staff.

My job offer came from Seaview Nursing and Residential Home situated in a commanding seafront position overlooking the promenade in Clacton. It was a family owned business and not part of a care home group, which obviously enabled increased flexibility when it came to staffing and terms, etc. The home manager was a dual qualified RGN/RMN called Mark. He, like many psychiatric trained nurse's I had met and worked with during my nurse training, had a very calm, likeable demeanour. He operated an extremely informal, yet effective style of management and as a family man with two children and a wife who was also a nurse working in the private sector in Colchester, he totally understood the flexibility needed to enable parents to work. More importantly for me was that he was one of the first people to introduce me to the importance of reflective practice as part of my continued professional development way ahead of its introduction to the private aged care establishments and businesses. From the start, Mark was keen to point out that there would be plenty of career enhancement and progression opportunities available to committed staff members.

Sarah Jane Butfield

I pride myself on the fact that whatever job or position I have held whether as a nurse, bar maid, cleaner or fruit picker, I have always given my total loyalty and commitment, so I felt confident that this position was an excellent fit for me, my career and most importantly my young family. I accepted the position of part time staff nurse working two, eight to ten hour shifts on the weekends and importantly earning more than I had working 30-36 hours' week as a care assistant. The downside of this arrangement was that Keith had to wake Samantha and Robert at 9.30pm to drive to Clacton to pick me up and then we had to settle our babies again when we got home. The tremendous upside however was that Monday to Friday I could be totally committed to being a stay at home mum and could invest time into my academic professional development, now that I worked in an aged care environment that presented knowledge and skill requirements that differed from my geriatric experiences in the NHS.

Being in charge soon felt normal, as the trained nurse routine revolved around care planning, allocation of tasks and duties, administering medication and wound care. Nursing home residents cover a varied clientele that became known as the aged care sector. Increasingly this description became both politically and physically incorrect as our residents included both males and females between the age of 18 and 100+. These poor souls with a variety of conditions and disabilities including, Parkinson's, Alzheimer's, arthritis and MS, could no longer physically cope or be cared for in their own homes. The pastoral care of spouses and extended family members, when you care for residents over such a large age range formed a major part of the nursing and caring role, regardless of whether the resident was in for respite or long term care. In the hospital setting, pastoral care focused on the patient and close family during the acute stages of their admission, and again during the discharge planning process. However, in the aged care setting this aspect of care provision took on a new perspective for healthcare workers of all grades. The biggest difference was that all grades of staff were actively involved in pastoral care and it was no longer just the remit of the qualified nurses.

Pastoral care can, and has, been described in a variety of ways over the years, often depending on how it is being applied. McKinlay, 2001 described it as *"being with people in a time of need to promote well-being while strengthening their spirituality."* Spiritual and pastoral care is often referred to as one and the same thing in healthcare reference books. However, spirituality alone was defined by Hunglemann, Kenkel- Rossi, Klassen, & Stollenwork, in 1985 as, *"connecting with one's self and others meaning God or higher powers."* This made sense in aged care because, in relation to older people, it was generally discussed in relation to their spiritual needs due to the lack of specific guidance about pastoral care in the aged care reference books.

The provision of pastoral care to an increasing elderly population was no longer seen as a recommended action, but a required vital element of the care of older people. Over the last ten years many countries, including Australia, where I have since worked as a qualified nurse, place a high emphasis on pastoral care. They address it by providing trained personnel specifically to identify and implement the pastoral care needs in all healthcare settings to benefit not only their patients but also their families, the healthcare staff and the local community. These specially trained staff work particularly closely with nurses, to provide the resources and support needed. However, I sometimes found it difficult to find information on how to provide high quality pastoral care in the aged care setting. Therefore, I made this a focus of my professional development. I believed that it played an enormous part in the way residents both settle into their new home and how their healthcare needs were accommodated in the longer term. Most of the evidence led research related to pastoral care would not take place until the late 1990s.

My pastoral care training and experience within the NHS, initially as a student nurse and later as a staff nurse working in geriatrics, was targeted on enabling spouses and family members to cope with acute, emergency changes to their loved one's physical and/or psychological condition either due to illness, accident or degenerative changes. The aim was to provide support during their stay and to help prepare the patient and their family for discharge home or to an appropriate healthcare setting. Even though I had taken part in discharge planning of patients going into aged care facilities for long term care when I worked on the medical and geriatric wards I realised, once I was working in aged care, how sometimes that preparation is far from adequate and I appreciated the importance that needs to be placed on pastoral care during the transition period. I now experienced feelings of guilt, in hindsight, at my ignorance when I had been working in the acute sector to the physical, emotional, psychological and social effects that a move to aged care takes on the patient and his/her family.

The move to an aged care facility is a huge decision and one that affects, and should involve, the patient/resident, their family and their network of friends, all of whom will play an integral part in the acceptance of the move. Although I believed that I understood the theoretical rationale and how to deal with the emotions and practical implications, I soon realised that all I knew was how to make the logistics of the move happen with little thought or attention to the pastoral care needed. Now as a staff nurse in a nursing home I admitted poorly prepared residents and their families from hospitals in the local area and I found that my pastoral care role initially involved a great deal of apologising for the lack of information, guidance and support given to them from the hospital staff in preparation for the enormity of the move to aged care.

This care of the spouses and the extended family of permanent and respite residents took on a deeper more emotional meaning. For many this was their first time in a nursing home and that alone could be daunting. There were many preconceived ideas about the types of people that we cared for, the disabilities they suffered from and the conditions in which they would be living. Over the next few months I worked hard to improve my knowledge and handling of this aspect of my role as it was very apparent that good pastoral care helped residents and their families enormously and in some cases improved their physical well-being. I enjoyed this work immensely.

The first couple of months with this new work life balance were exhilarating. I had energy, no night duties meant quality sleep despite still breast feeding Robert and I even managed to get back to regular exercising to regain my pre-pregnancy figure. The work as the weekend late shift staff nurse was also fulfilling. I administered medications and dealt with acute onset illness and accidents. I assisted the care staff with pressure area care, toileting, bedtime routines and interacted with family and friends of the relatives. I quickly became involved with the hands-on teaching and education of the care staff as the staff turnover was high and so basic personal care skills always needed to be taught.

One Saturday I arrived 30 minutes early for my late shift, as normal, because I liked to have the time and opportunity to read the communications book to catch up on the changes since my last shift the previous weekend. On the late shift, I as always in-charge, but Mark was contactable for emergencies or professional advice. Mark lived nearby which was reassuring as he never hesitated to offer to come and assist or assess if a resident fell or became acutely ill and needed a doctor's visit or hospital attendance. He would often pop in at the weekend with his two young daughters, sometimes on roller-skates if they had been skating on the promenade, just to check all was well.

After reading the communications book I made my way to the back room that we used for the staff handover meetings, training, etc. There would always be a tray of tea laid out ready by the morning staff for us to drink during handover. As I entered the room I noticed a white envelope with my name on it beside the tray, I poured my tea and sat down to read the contents. The typewritten, short letter inside congratulated me on being promoted to the position of Deputy Matron, which sounded odd as Mark was always referred to as the home manager not the matron. What had brought about the development of this new position? How had I been selected without any formal application or interview process? Who cared! I felt honoured, respected and over joyed that my nursing and management skills had been noticed and were now being recognised in the form of a promotion.

I called Keith and explained what had happened. He listened without saying much and most disappointingly he didn't congratulate me. I was excited to talk to Mark about how we would work together as an influx of plans and ideas flooded my head. These included ways I could use my new position and role to enhance care provision and be a suitably able support to the manager and the owners. I decided not to dwell on the lack of interest during my telephone conversation with Keith as I felt sure we would continue the discussion in more detail later. I had probably caught him at a bad moment, after all he did have a toddler and a baby to care for. My excitement was short lived as later that afternoon I discovered that Mark was no longer employed at Seaview Nursing Home and in the short-term I was in charge! Professional anxiety and self-doubt about being able to even temporarily fill his shoes with only the support of the owners crept in. However, the staff were all congratulating me, but also gossiping about what may, or may not, have happened to result in the sudden, unexplained exit of Mark, and that left little time to reflect or worry, I just had to get on with it.

The home owners called me at home on the Monday morning and explained that Mark had resigned due to personal reasons and that he had no opportunity to work his notice. Therefore, they would be grateful if I could step in and address as many managerial tasks as possible during my weekend shifts if they employed another qualified nurse to work with me to free up time for these activities. I accepted the position, and their explanation, and I looked forward to going into work the following Saturday to get started. I didn't need to wait that long. By Wednesday the telephone had been ringing daily with staff wanting to talk to me about the next fortnights staff rota and the owners wanting to alert me to medication supply issues that they needed resolving with the pharmacy, etc. I discussed and agreed with Keith that I would go into work for a nine to five management shift on Thursday, travelling by bus so that Keith could still go to work and my good friend Sue could babysit for us.

The office based shift was incredible. I realised I knew so much more than I had first imagined. I was able to resolve the staff rota issues to accommodate the needs of a couple of the single mums who were having trouble juggling their childcare and shift patterns. I discussed the medication issues with the pharmacist and had the local doctor's surgery reissue the medication chart to avoid future confusion. As much as I thoroughly enjoyed working hands on with our residents and staff I knew that I could get used to a managerial position very easily, but it was early days and I was letting my head runaway with ideas of professional grandeur. Reality struck that evening when I got home. Keith had collected the children from Sue and was sat in the dark in the lounge with just the television on and the children playing in front of it. I switched the light on and hugged the children and looked across at Keith. He was clearly sulking.

"Did you have a bad day?" I asked, a little disappointed that he showed no signs of enquiring about my first day in a managerial role.

"This is not happening again, ok?" Was all he said, before grabbing his coat and heading out of the front door.

This would be the beginning of the end of our marriage, as little by little, events and people became involved that tore apart the foundations of our relationship which had been in place since I was 16 years old. Naively, I had no idea what the long-term ramifications of this would be for me emotionally. 'Ignorance is bliss,' they say, and 'Hindsight is wonderful thing.' Both are true, but it is of little consolation after the event.

Chapter Six: New skills needed

My new promotion brought with it new roles, responsibilities and opportunities that I had previously only observed in my senior peer group both in the NHS and at Cheviot Nursing and Residential Home. Now it was my turn to take the lead in the training and education of the care assistants in our team. The aim was to equip them with knowledge and practical skills to enable them to deliver high standards of personal care, focusing on the health and safety of not only the residents, but also themselves and the other care and nursing staff. Moving and handling, which was simply called 'lifting' back then, was a major problem for the small, independent homes with limited access to mobile and fixed lifting apparatus, hoists and mobility aids. Added to this was the fact that Seaview, like many other old buildings that were converted into nursing and residential homes, was in places impractical and unfit for purpose with narrow, twisting corridors and winding staircases. Workplace injuries, back strains and occasionally falls and incidents involving residents were a big problem because it impacted on sickness absences, staffing levels and on the nursing homes reputation.

Over the years, I had heard many horror stories from healthcare staff of all grades who had experienced, or knew someone who had, a back or neck injury sustained whilst moving a resident or a piece of their equipment. I knew all too well that a back injury could end your nursing career, unless you were high ranking with additional skillsets that added value to the healthcare sector. However, many care assistants, who often had no sense of value for the service they supplied, seemed prepared to take unnecessary risks with their own personal safety and that of the residents they were caring for. Overcoming this mind-set was one of the biggest hurdles when it came to training them. I liked to take a hands-on approach and teach them to appreciate what it feels like to be a resident by using role play. I would ask them to practice on one another, sometimes strapping limbs together to imitate restricted ability and to stop the staff from trying to help when they were being moved. When I had been a participant in this kind of role play, it was always a big reality check to experience the lack of control of your own limbs and to fully appreciate the fear that this induced for our residents. I constantly referred to methods, case studies and rationale taught to me during my student nurse training as I truly believed that quality training could and would make a difference.

Of course, I met a great deal of resistance from some of the older care assistants who had been operating with bad practices for years and who, despite many of them openly complaining about back pain, strains and health issues, blatantly refused to carry out the safe practices I taught them. Some of them were very over weight which added to their personal risk factors.

Bedpans to Boardrooms

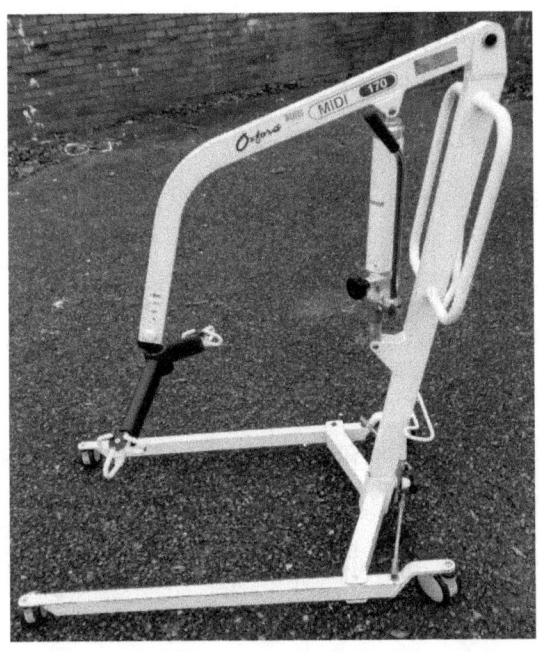

At Seaview, we had a small Oxford hoist for residents on the first floor and it had a weight carrying limit of up to about 18 - 20 stone, (114 to 127 kg), but it never looked as if it could accommodate anyone of that size! We used to weigh our residents every week on a Sunday and keep a book to record the information, partly so that we knew if they were safe to be transferred in the equipment we had within the home and whether they needed a transfer to the ground floor. As the larger hoists had to be on the ground floor due to the corridor size this meant only the lighter residents could be accommodated on the 1st floor. In the same vein, we had to weigh the care assistants before we could let them take part in the hoist training practical elements. It was during one of these training sessions that three staff were unable to take part in the role play as residents because they were too heavy to be hoisted, started to realise what this could mean that if they were taken ill. There could be the possibility of them not getting the care they needed if bariatric moving equipment was not available.

Bariatric is a term which was not widely used at that time, but is prevalent nowadays due to the increase in obesity based medicine and healthcare requirements. The term Bariatric means, 'a branch of medicine that deals with the prevention, causes and treatment of obesity and its complications'. Bariatric equipment is large, mechanically reinforced versions of mobility and nursing aids for obese patients. The range includes commodes, hoists, chairs and weighing scales, which had added width, depth and strength. Anyway, I digress, back to our over-weight care assistants! The positive outcome from their slightly embarrassing withdrawal from the practical lifting training was that they decided to do something proactive about their size and they started a Weight Watchers slimming group.

They held their meetings in the resident's lounge on a Tuesday evening when the residents had retired to their rooms. The group became very successful with several stones in weight being lost by its members. This had a massive impact on the staff morale not just because they could now take part with everyone else, but the better they felt about themselves the happier they became in the work place. A wave of willingness to achieve more, both personally and professionally, swept through the nursing home as the staff of all grades started to take a proactive interest in the health and wellbeing of themselves and our residents.

In teaching basic personal care, skills such as bed baths, washing hair in bed, pressure area care and hygiene and dealing with incontinence are all essential skills. With a team of care staff who ranged in age from 16 - 66 it was obvious from the outset that the education and training could not be a 'one size fits all'. The staff who were parents, or who had cared for elderly relatives of their own, had a head start with the practical side of things. However, teaching the young, inexperienced staff was easier in that they had no preconceived ideas to fall back on so they readily adopted the procedures and skills which they were taught like learning to drive. As they practiced alongside proficient care staff and other trained nurses they became more thorough and capable of reporting their observations of skin integrity, changes to bowel or urination habits and feeding difficulties. All of this helped to improve the level of care provided throughout the home. We had a strong team ethos growing and the positive energy it produced became infectious throughout the home amongst residents and staff.

Who wants to be a care assistant?

When I trained to be a nurse we had two male students in our group. Later, when I was working as a care assistant in Brightlingsea there were no male staff apart from the home owners. Working in Clacton it was a totally different story. At Seaview Nursing Home, as you know, the previous manager was a male dual trained RGN/RMN and although most of the qualified nurses were female, the proportion of males amongst the care assistants was increasing, with more men coming into the aged care sector out of choice and due to increased local job availability.

At a time when career and social expectations prior to this period had been that care assistants and nurses should, and would, be female, this changing trend was difficult for some of the residents to accept, particularly the female ones. I found myself working in aged care due to my family commitments, a need for part time, flexible hours and for financial reasons. For male, qualified nurses, possibly the main bread winners in their family, the move to aged care may not have been a first choice as it could have been perceived as career limiting. However, the opportunity for a salary higher than that offered in the local NHS was appealing. For male care assistants, who upskilled with in-house training and who worked a basic 40-hour week they too achieved a good wage compared to other local industries and so the aged care opportunities became lucrative propositions. Young men and women with no qualifications were limited in their job searches by the access and restrictions provided by public transport in relation to working shifts therefore, the straight from school 16 - 18 year olds from Clacton quickly became the backbone of the staffing in many of the local nursing and residential homes. For young men who did not want to work on a building site or on one of the many local holiday parks, as Clacton was a popular seaside town, the aged care sector offered many opportunities both in care and ancillary service provision. The other group of male staff were older men, semi-retired, wanting to earn some money, but also wanting to contribute to their local community. This combination of age, energy, experience and enthusiasm boosted the impact of having a growing male contingent, and some of the male residents loved it. The other large group of staff were young mums seeking part time work and women approaching retirement who needed flexibility. These two groups of women brought with them experience as parents and as care assistants, but also logistical and managerial issues such as childcare provision and bad habits from previous aged care employment.

The course I had been completing as part of my professional development had helped me to develop the skillset and confidence to push for high standards of care provision from the staff that I managed, but the issue of retaining them was a competitive and complex one. Clacton at that time was renowned for being the 'home hoppers paradise'. Nursing and residential homes would invest heavily to provide in-house and external training, which at the time was only a recommendation and not a requirement of the licensing authorities.

More homes were opening in Clacton and in other seaside towns and villages and the staff that became well trained could command higher rates of pay to stay or be enticed away by other homes. Some staff would leave and then want to return when they realised that the glittering promises made at interview often didn't materialise. Care assistants who had been well trained in enhanced level of care provision now felt compromised in poor working environments and would not overlook poor standards or questionable unsafe working practices in other homes. For this reason, they soon became sort after by homes that were struggling with accreditation or that had been put on notice to improve.

I soon became experienced at spotting the new arrivals who were eager to participate quickly in the free training, especially activities that were certified and who would then disappear with their certificates, often with no notice, to a neighbouring nursing or residential home. Once the in-house training had been established we decided to introduce a range of staff incentives to retain our valued staff. These included flexible working, split shifts to accommodate school hours and even our own in-house crèche. There was no quick fix solution to the staffing dilemma faced by all the local homes, but it was crucial for each home to find it's unique selling point not just to attract new residents and achieve full occupancy, but also to attract good, reliable staff who would uphold the values and ethos of the home. Staffing was always an agenda item at the monthly local authority, home manager meetings where we would supposedly share ideas on recruitment, retention and training. However, as the competition for staff increased many home owners and managers became guarded in their participation in these discussions for fear of losing the upper hand. The sharing of best practice was a new concept in this arena at the time, but one that would be developed and nurtured in a range of fields relative to aged care over the next five to ten years.

Chapter Seven: Consequences and compromises

"For every action, there is an equal and opposite reaction." Newton's Third Law.

The harsh truth and stark reality of this statement became apparent to me within a few months of supposedly resurrecting my career. After my almost grieving for my floundering nursing career whilst working as a care assistant in Brightlingsea, out of necessity and convenience, my career had now been kick-started with my promotion to the position of Deputy Matron. Within a short period of time that gave us some much needed financial stability to help support our growing family. When we achieve goals, dreams or ambitions in life, that bring us happiness and appears to solve our problems. However, as we all know, other problems or challenges can, and will, develop. I was totally to blame for the events that followed as I allowed myself to become self-absorbed with my work, my new colleagues and the freedom that our improved finances permitted.

A few months later and it was all change as I now found myself living as a single mum with two small children in the flat above the nursing home after the slow and painful breakup of my marriage. This new living arrangement was totally outside my comfort zone, but not because I was a single mum for the first time, because I always felt confident in caring and being fully responsible for my children 24/7. It was more because, apart from my time living in the nurses' quarters during my nurse training, this was the first time I had lived alone, well apart from having two little ones in tow! The benefits of this new arrangement were that I had no commute to work other than two flights of stairs, which was formally known as the fire exit! My childcare was taking place in the flat I now rented as part of my salary package. The childcare shifts were shared between two good friends I had made, Michelle and Vicky, who were also care assistants at Seaview. During the troubled few months prior to my separation from Keith they had listened, supported and kept me focused on finding the balance between family and career. However, I chose to dress up this drastic change in my personal circumstances, I was making a huge sacrifice with massive risk, and sometimes I wondered, 'For what?' There will be times later in this book when you will question, as I did with the benefit of hindsight, if it was worth it. In the short term is was a massive risk, but in the very long term eventually I hoped it would be worth it.

I was financially secure working full-time as the nurse in charge of the home and I worked, safe in the knowledge that Samantha and Robert were well cared for in the same building. I knew that if I was needed I could be with them in minutes. Samantha and Robert were thoroughly spoilt by all the staff at the home. Whenever I was on a break either Vicky or Michelle would bring them down to see me and when there was entertainment on for the residents they would also attend. They loved the visiting church and Salvation Army choirs and the local school children that came in. As we lived literally opposite the promenade Vicky and Michelle would take them for a seaside walk every day. It was like a permanent holiday for them, playing on the beach, running around and generally having fun. I did regret my lack of time with them, but my work load was increasing with the responsibility I now held. The owners had long since stopped trying to replace Mark as they now had me living on site performing both roles. It was still a good financial deal for me though because I was earning a good salary with very few overheads. As I compiled the staff rosters I had a degree of flexibility and so when Samantha started nursery school I made sure I could take her and pick her up, just one of the parenting experiences that I would not be compromising on.

It all worked perfectly, maybe too perfectly at times, and looking back, I think I took my eye off the ball in relation to my personal life. I invested all my free time into my professional development courses being eager to return to acute care nursing one day. As much as I loved the day to day work with the elderly and infirm, and while I enjoyed the thrill of dealing with in-house emergencies, including falls, sudden onset illness such as heart attacks, respiratory distress and other comorbidities of chronic disease, but this wasn't where I envisaged my career going. The harder I studied to stay up to date with best practice, techniques etc. the more I aspired to achieving an acute care position in the future. I found a way to add some practical acute care experience to my nursing portfolio by joining the BNA (British Nursing Association). Nursing agencies cover temporary shifts in hospitals, clinics, nursing homes and in the community. I could only manage one shift a month as I had to be able to travel to Colchester for the work by public transport and I was keen that most my time off was spent with Samantha and Robert, but for six hours once a month the agency shift gave me my acute care fix.

The skillset and management courses I was completing gave me the confidence to push for better facilities and higher staffing levels for our residents. However, it was a tough balancing act because the owners didn't want to invest in this, but the staff needed to see a benefit for the extra work and learning involved in change management. The management role at Seaview Nursing Home was developing into a very diverse nursing role, and by far one of the most time-consuming tasks was staff recruitment, training and retention. With our staffing at Seaview stabilising and with full occupancy plus a waiting list in place it was not long before numerous offers to buy the nursing home as a going concern started to arrive from the national nursing home groups. The owners of Seaview turned down many lucrative deals, but the face of the nursing home business was changing and nursing home reforms were on the cards.

Little did I know at the time, as I was not well versed in due diligence methods, that checks and investigations were being carried out by the national care home providers before they acquired homes. As part of this they checked for qualified staffing levels both in the nursing home they were targeting and in the local area. It became common practice that visitors to nursing and residential homes came under the pretence of looking for accommodation for elderly or infirm relatives, but their questioning was more focused on the staff and their credential's than on the home's facilities. This information was freely given as it was crucial to be transparent and to show off your staffing expertise. Selling beds and achieving that one hundred percent full occupancy status was a key part of the management role and 'walk-ins', particularly on weekends, were a regular occurrence. The guided tour of the home would be followed by up to an hour of questions and answers. The provision of a glossy brochure with its mission statement and overview of the home's ethos was the final parting gift, but never revealing the pricing, as mystery shoppers from other nursing and residential homes also used this tactic to find out the going rates in homes so that they could price match or undercut. This was my first taste of selling within the nursing profession and it did not come naturally. However, I was very proud of the nursing, care and ancillary teams that I worked with and I had no problem singing their praises to prospective residents and their families. As a result of their due diligence exercises the national care home providers built up 'hot lists' of homes for possible acquisition and qualified staff to target with job proposals. Gossip in the nursing home community was rife. A hot bed of Chinese whispers about the happenings in other homes, their staff and work practices, circulated, even down to discussing the menus! It was crucial for home owners, matrons and managers to keep abreast of the gossip in case there were elements of truth to be gleaned.

The accountable manager, or person in charge, also appeared on a register held by the local council and authorities. The qualifications, background police record checks and professional references were checked regularly for compliance with local and national codes of conduct and practice. This was in addition to the requirements of the national nursing registration boards. Quality Assurance was on the way in and would become the buzz word in the aged care sector over the next two to three years.

As the Deputy Matron at Seaview I was now on the radar of the both the local and national care home providers and it wasn't long before offers from head hunters started. I was initially flattered, but also wary of why they would have any interest in someone with relatively limited time and experience in the aged care sector. I was lacking in confidence at this time due to the short period that I had worked in the sector and due to my personal relationship issues. The thought of moving out of what had now become my comfort zone was not appealing. I had a very good personal and professional life at Seaview with stability for myself as a single mum and my two small children. To go and see if the grass was greener on the other side would be a massive leap of faith. However, in

1991 things started to change for me personally. I had managed to maintain an amicable arrangement with Keith for contact with the children and we even enjoyed family days out together. I had a career pathway developing which I was pursuing with vigour and I had my acute care studies and practical shifts to aim for an acute care nursing position maybe when Samantha and Robert both reached school age. But I was lonely. It sounds silly to say or write those words as I was surrounded by staff, friends and residents who I adored, but I needed more. It is not an excuse, or maybe it is, but I let my loneliness cloud my judgement when a charming male care assistant began working at Seaview. However, having a relationship with a member of staff when you 'live above the shop' as they say in Essex was never going to work and I realised that it was time to find a home of my own away from work so that I could start to think about starting again in a new relationship.

I looked for houses to rent near to the children's nursery school, but still within walking distance of work. The owners of Seaview tried to change my mind, reassuring me that personal and professional lives could be maintained with privacy and dignity in the current living arrangements. I doubted that and as my house search continued it was not long before the news of my plan to live off site soon became a topic of the local gossip.

Chapter Eight: A new home, a new relationship and ultimately a new job!

I never intended, nor would I ever advise anyone to attempt to make three high risk, life changing events happen within weeks of each other, but it was happening and regardless of the timing I now had to make it work for me and the children. What I wanted, and needed, most from this new combination of life and career events was to focus on the future and to find happiness and fulfilment in both my personal and professional life. However, what I managed to find was heartbreak, confusion and frustration.

As a single mum now embarking on the first serious relationship since the breakup of my marriage I really should have been more careful. In hindsight, I should have listened to the warnings from my friends, colleagues and family members who could see from the outside what was happening. The painful truth is that I was flattered by the attention of a charming man five years younger than me who started work at Seaview. His name was Jack. The fact that he was the local Casanova should have made me step well away, but quite the reverse was true. It made me feel special because he seemingly preferred a woman with two children and some relationship baggage, to any of the younger, prettier girls with no ex-husbands or children to deal with. I let this man into the life of myself and my children and far too quickly we moved in together. Within a few months, with my work life ticking all the boxes for me, we even started talking about buying a house and having a child of our own. It was all too fast, but a mind-set of my needing to do whatever he wanted me to, in order to keep him happy, set it.

I became a victim and this made me accept behaviour from him that I never dreamed I was capable of. He would disappear for days on end, claiming to be visiting sick friends in London or to be on a car buying trip with his friend who owned a car sales lot in Colchester. My naïve acceptance didn't stop the arguments and rows we had when he returned from his unexpected, unexplained absences, but the manipulation of my emotions and mind-set meant that I did nothing to extract myself or my children from the situation. I know now it was initially the money from my divorce settlement that attracted him to me and after that a situation of I don't want her full time, but I don't want anyone else to have her developed. He fuelled this behaviour with his sob story about his strong desire to become a dad after being denied access to a son he had when he was younger. I fell for it thinking it would make him stay and settle down properly. When I became pregnant again everything changed for a while, he no longer stayed out late or disappeared. He cooked dinner for when I returned from work. He started to take a more hands on role with Samantha and Robert and I truly believed that this would be our happy ever after.

Bedpans to Boardrooms

On Valentine's Day, I returned home and he had the table laid for a candle-lit romantic dinner for two, which was cooking in the kitchen. The children were bathed and ready for bed in their pyjamas. He told me to go and read them a story, and settle them, then we could celebrate our first proper Valentine's Day together. I changed out of my uniform and spent some time settling the children. When they were asleep I was walking downstairs when a pain struck as if I had been stabbed. I cried out as I looked down and saw dark red blood dripping onto the beige stairs carpet. Jack called 999 and then Vicky to come and sit with the children. An ambulance arrived and I remember being lifted into it, but I don't really remember much else until I awoke at the hospital with Jack, his brother and his wife beside me. I knew I had lost the baby by the expressions on their faces and as I looked across at Jack I was sure that he would be the next loss I would experience.

True to form within a week Jack was gone and to be honest initially I didn't care. I was on sick leave from work following the miscarriage and I had time to reflect on some of the behaviours I had been tolerating from him and I had to ask myself the question, why? What did he add to my life? The simple answer was, absolutely nothing. He gave up work at Seaview when we moved in together claiming that he wanted to get to know the children by spending more time with them. This negated one of the reasons for me moving out of Seaview. I had become his meal ticket while he continued to claim the dole for being out of work. I bought him a new car, clothes and jewellery when he claimed to have lost everything to a vindictive ex-partner, which turned out to be a lie. I had been acting a fool, and taken for one and I convinced myself that I deserved it for the terrible way I behaved before the breakdown of my marriage to Keith. I became increasingly unsettled and when I returned to work the gossip about my personal life was intense. I knew the only course of action was to change my job and move out of Clacton. I needed to be somewhere that was familiar, and I also wanted to make sure that I used the remaining money from my divorce settlement to provide a stable home for Samantha and Robert.

With my professional experience, skills and reputation acquired at Seaview proudly displayed on my CV it was easy for me to find a new role as a deputy matron in Colchester. In 1992, Hill House, was a privately-owned nursing and residential home in the suburb of Lexden, opposite the maternity hospital where I had given birth to Samantha and Robert. I had no problem finding a lovely end terraced three-bedroom house near North Station which was near to the hospital where I worked my agency shifts and near to Mill Road where I lived in the nurse quarters when I first arrived in Colchester. It felt like returning home and I had a good feeling that this time everything would be alright.

A new chapter in my aged care journey was about to open, now all I needed was for it to run parallel to the changes in my personal life? My mum and my sisters had witnessed the catalogue of poor personal life decisions I had been making over the last two years and I think they were relieved when I showed signs of sorting myself out. The staff at Hill House were wonderful to work with and I soon felt as if I had worked there and been part of the team for years. The owner, Gillian, was a medically retired SRN (State Registered Nurse) and although most of the time she herself was confined to a wheelchair, she still had the knack of being able to negotiate her way through the home, which was formerly a Georgian manor house, to the staffroom to catch out care assistants and nurses who were taking extended breaks or sneaking out for a crafty cigarette. I was a regular attendee at the care home manager meetings in Colchester and I managed to extend and expand my knowledge of the care home industry, by networking with managers, matrons and deputies from a wide variety of homes.

Colchester was home to some of the national care home groups' and this was my first taste of the divide that existed between small and large homes. I am not referring to the physical properties here, although in the main the groups homes had 40 plus beds. Instead it was the manner and ethos that the managerial staff from these homes' brought to the table. Firstly, as they did not own the homes they had less of a personal, emotional attachment to the home. That is not to say they cared any less, or did not display their emotions, if their homes or staff were in any way criticised or needed defending. The private home owners tended to moan a little more especially if physical changes to the property were discussed or proposed as straight away the pound signs and the pull on their purse strings would appear. Secondly, the level of reporting and methods of approval needed for the group homes seemed to me, with no experience of it, like a hindrance to achieving change. This personal observation was of course due to my ignorance of the hierarchy and allocation of spending power from the boardroom down to the local home level at that time.

With my work life back on track and Samantha and Robert settled into new nursery and childcare placements I resumed my professional development studies and focused on learning some nurse management skills to complement my role. I continued to work my acute care agency shifts, one or twice a month, and everything was going well until the afternoon of 26th November 1992. I was in a staff meeting at work with the other qualified nurses discussing changes to the ordering and storing of medications. We were interrupted by the nursing home's secretary, Rebecca, who said she had an urgent telephone call that I needed to take. Immediately I presumed that one of the children had been hurt, or was ill, so I rushed to the office. I remember standing listening to the voice on the telephone, but not really taking in the content after the initial words, 'It's about your mother'. I remember dropping the telephone receiver, leaving it dangling on its coiled wire, and running to collect my handbag. I came to a sudden halt at the back door with tears running down my face as I realised I had no way to get to Ipswich Hospital quickly, and I would need someone to pick up Samantha and Robert later and look after them until I returned. A strong, reassuring hand descended onto my shoulder, gripping me tightly. It was Ron, the co-owner of the home and Gillian's ex-husband. He offered to drive me and said that Rebecca and Gillian would make the necessary arrangements for the children.

Mum had not been well over the years, she suffered with heart problems and had previously had a stroke, but she always just kept going. She was on warfarin tablets to thin her blood, but that didn't stop her developing a pulmonary embolism. I didn't arrive in time to say goodbye properly and I have so many words that are still unsaid. Life can be cruel, I did, and still do, need and miss my mum and at 56 years old she was taken from us far too soon, before seeing and knowing how her children went on to have many more beautiful grandchildren, and now great grandchildren.

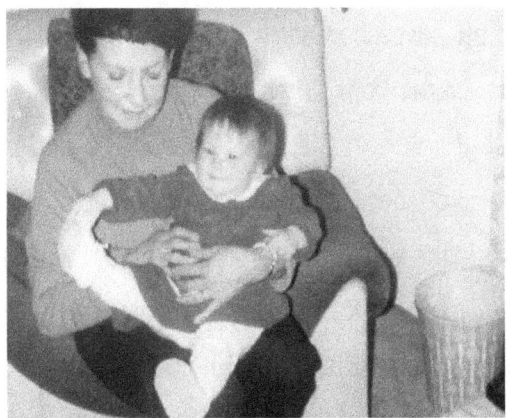

My mum with Samantha, one of the precious grandchildren she did meet.

Chapter Nine: All change!

Jack had not completely disappeared from my life since my move to Colchester, but somehow up until now his behaviour, which hadn't changed, didn't upset me quite as much. Maybe I had hardened myself to it. That all changed early in 1993 when I allowed him back into my home and our lives again. He had a full-time job as a care assistant and he seemed to be distancing himself from the people he had previously associated with in Clacton. I was beginning to feel trapped in my job as there was nothing to inspire any ambition. There would never be a position to be promoted to because Gillian was the Matron and she owned the home. We didn't have a high turnover of residents so there was rarely anything new or medically exciting to get my teeth into. So when I spotted an advertisement in the local paper for a Senior Sister position at The Carnarvon Nursing Home, offering daytime shifts it sounded ideal, but it was in Clacton. Transport to and from work would be easy as we lived near the railway station in Colchester, and the Clacton railway station was less than a five-minute walk from the nursing home. The train journey was only 25 minutes so it was all possible without relying on Jack for anything. But could I really step back into the nursing home circuit in Clacton? What would be my motivation? Well at this point in my aged care career, for me it was the appeal of working for a national care home group, with the structure that I initially observed as a hindrance offering my career a future, as I seem destined to remain in aged care.

Within a few days of my interview a formal job offer arrived. It was not a management role, which initially took the shine off, because I did enjoy the management aspects of my roles at Seaview and Hill House. However, the clinical appeal for me, from the nursing perspective, was that a larger home, which also offered convalescence and respite care placements to more acute care residents, would mean increased opportunities to utilise the 'real' nursing skills that I loved and missed. In addition to the fact that it was still within the aged care sector. It was a 'win, win,' situation. They offered flexible, daytime working hours to accommodate childcare needs and proposed company funding of an accredited course to formalise the skills needed for the teaching care assistants. This was something that I had been carrying out for the last year or so informally. This was a big draw for me as I enjoyed teaching practical skills and to be able to learn how to format lessons, plan handouts and deliver training workshops, funded by the company, was an excellent opportunity.

I accepted the offer of a Senior Sister position reporting directly to the home manager, Annette Needham. I was still a form of deputy, but with a different title, at least that's how I liked to think of it as there were no other nursing or management positions in the operational structure between the four senior sisters and the home manager.

Sarah Jane Butfield

The Carnarvon Nursing Home was owned by the national care home group Associated Nursing Services (ANS). Their head office was based at their flagship nursing home Meadbank in Battersea, London. The Carnarvon Nursing Home occupied a grand building which was built in the late 1800s when the town developed with the arrival of the paddle steamer industry and the building of the railway connecting Clacton to London. The home occupied the houses of 22 – 24 Carnarvon Road. Before being converted into a nursing home it was a grand hotel and, like many others in the town that undertook the same conversion to a nursing or residential home, it was ideally situated within walking distance of the town centre, the railway station and the seafront.

As I stepped into my new role as a Senior Sister working for a private national care home group for the first time there were immediate differences to the set up and environmental conditions for both staff and residents which overall were positive. A benefit from a qualified nurse perspective was that many of the aspects of care delivery were heavily documented and bureaucratic. This was similar to working in the NHS, whereas in the smaller privately owned homes where I had begun my aged care nursing journey, documented procedures were much less obvious or enforced. Although initially daunting to get to grips with, the documentation was not a bad thing and the accountability and evidence trail was something that I found immediately reassuring. I quickly realised I had missed this element of professionalism since leaving the NHS. I began to scrutinise the events that had occurred in my professional capacity as a nurse during my time at Seaview and Hill House and to think about areas where I may have been exposed professionally through ignorance of the aged care system, but I believed I had acted well and within the guidelines to date even if the evidence trail was limited.

The term 'Aged Care' can conjure up a variety of images depending on your age and life experiences, but some stereotypical ones may consist of grey hair, Zimmer frames, wheelchairs and some form of physical or psychological impairment. People who can longer care for themselves, or be cared for by family or support services at home, fall into this category. Nursing, residential and rest homes became big business during this period as did care in the community and respite care for younger adults with chronic disease or life limiting conditions.

It was not until I started working at The Carnarvon that I first cared for a new category of residents classified as YCS, meaning Young Chronically Sick. These were male and female residents, aged between 18-60 years. The conditions, disorders and disabilities that made them part of this group included MS (Multiple Sclerosis), MD (Muscular Dystrophy), Rheumatoid Arthritis and accident trauma victims, for example from road traffic accidents, workplace falls, horse riding accidents, to name but a few. Some convalescent care cases, where the residents fell into this age group, for example post-operative orthopaedic procedures, were the most common temporary addition to this group. The approach to caring for young chronically sick residents, with an array of medical, personal and social care needs, including physical, emotional, psychological and pastoral care involved a whole new skill-set and presented a range of challenges that, in my career to date, I had not encountered.

Some of these young residents were permanent, but a large majority came in on regular, respite placements. The reasons for their respite placements were varied, but the commonest was the need for their carers to have regular, well-deserved physical and psychological breaks from 24/7 caring. The importance of respite care packages for the carer as well as the resident was increasingly being researched and recommended by GP's and rehabilitation consultants as a way of helping to maintain care for young chronically sick people in the community by family and community allied healthcare professional teams. Respite care for residents needing access to specialised equipment for lifting or feeding meant these beds were always full and pre-booked. Occasionally residents would come in for assessment by the community allied healthcare professionals to facilitate changes to their nursing care plan that needed close observation before being managed solely in the community. For example, they might need assistance with medication changes or new mobility equipment and devices. In addition, nursing homes also had practical resources such as King's Fund, hospital style beds, which at that time were almost nonexistent for care in the community and were particularly useful for convalescent post-operative residents. More advanced and efficient lifting and mobility aids were available within the home with suitably qualified staff to implement the use of them. In addition, access to resources from other allied healthcare departments such as physiotherapy and occupational therapy were provided.

The young chronically sick became a specialist yet broad term for a variety of chronic diseases and conditions that presented with physical or mental disability and/or some form of self-care impairment. Little did I know at this stage that this field of nursing would become a big part of my career in the future. It was the high demand for this type of care in this age group which led to a large investment by ANS in which I would play a creative part, but more of that later.

Another group of residents that occasionally crossed the age barrier were EMI meaning Elderly, Mentally, Impaired, (formerly Infirm) These were younger residents, who didn't fit the 'elderly' criteria of EMI care, who needed respite and long term care for conditions such as early onset Alzheimer's, dementia, Parkinson's Disease or as a result of head injury. The youngest person that I cared for in the aged care setting was 33! This was an unnerving experience being in my twenties and with my ex-husband and father of my children 11 years my senior. It brought home to me the vulnerability of life and how an accident, illness or incident can change every aspect of daily life in a variety of ways and not just physically.

"Linda", a 33-year-old mother of two young girls fell from a horse. Initially there were no obvious injuries apart from a slight concussion and headache. She was discharged home after 48 hours of observation in hospital, however a few days later she was found collapsed at home with a sub acute, subdural hematoma, a serious medical condition where a collection of blood occurs between the skull and the surface of the brain, usually as a result of a direct trauma head injury. The symptoms can include

persistent headache

nausea and vomiting

mental confusion

mood swings and changed personality traits, for example aggressive behaviour and verbal outbursts, etc.

extreme, sudden drowsiness

In severe cases, there can be a loss of consciousness

Any or all of these symptoms can develop spontaneously following a severe head injury, when the illness is known as an acute subdural haematoma. Or they can develop a few days or weeks after a seemingly minor head injury, which is known as a sub acute or chronic subdural haematoma.

Linda required surgery to drain the haematoma, which was completed successfully. However, she was left with impaired mobility, short term memory loss and behavioural issues. Her husband and young family were unable to cope at home despite community support and Linda became a long stay resident at The Carnarvon.

Until the 1990s there was little provision or specialised care available for people aged 18 - 55 who for a variety of reasons needed full time care, attention and/or medical supervision, which for one reason or another could not be supported permanently in their own homes. There is a range of issues that the young chronically sick face when they must be cared for in an aged care setting which I will elaborate on in the upcoming chapters.

In the hospital setting when acute nursing care, observation and specialist therapies no longer need medical interventions, the hospital discharge teams will work with community healthcare teams to facilitate the patients discharge to free up the expensive hospital bed and associated staffing. The first assessment to be made is to establish if the young person is able to return to their own home and if so what adaptions, equipment and support services, if appropriate, they will need.

There are various reasons and barriers to making this happen which include:

Qualified medical assistance is needed for medication, therapy and feeding.

Care assistant skills are needed to enable the daily living activities to be performed, i.e., toileting, personal hygiene, feeding, etc.

The patient's home environment is not suitable for their needs – size of doorways, steps and access from outdoors, toilet and bathroom layout, stairs, etc.

Lack of equipment required for the safe performance of daily activities, such as a hoist or pressure area care mattress/aids, etc.

When a patient was assessed in hospital as fit for discharge, pending community care support, then it was the role of the social work and allied healthcare teams to put together a package of care and equipment to enable a move back to their home environment. However, in some cases this was not practical or possible and these young people would be placed on a waiting list for a bed in aged care facility. Ideally it would be one that had a specialist unit, staff and support services aimed at care provision for young people or one that demonstrated an ethos of care that recognised the special physical, psychological and medical needs of this group of residents. Funding for either the home adaptions needed and regular respite care packages if a move to home was feasible or the funding of long term care was governed by legislation originating in 1970 with The Chronically Sick and Disabled Persons Act which:

"Placed a duty of care on all local authorities to make arrangements for the provision of assistance for an eligible disabled person for adaptations to the home, or the provision of any additional facilities designed to secure greater safety, comfort or convenience. This also includes the provision of equipment and welfare services."

The non-medical support may seem basic, but nonetheless it was vital to the success of a home care package. Here is an excerpt from the Act in relation to services and facilities to be provided:

"Practical assistance in the home;

Provision (or assistance to obtain) radio, TV, library or other recreational services;

Provision of lectures, games, outings, recreational or educational activities outside the home;

Provision of services or assistance in obtaining travel to and from the home to participate in any of the activities mentioned;

> *Assistance in arranging adaptations or provision of additional facilities to promote "safety, comfort or convenience";*
>
> *Provision of meals in the home or elsewhere;*
>
> *Assistance in obtaining a phone and any special equipment necessary to use it."*

Such was the extent of care provision expected for the chronically sick or disabled and a similar standard was expected in care homes.

My return to a more predominantly nursing role with access to residents with a wider variation of diseases, disorders and disabilities helped me to refocus my professional education to more medically relevant topics. We had a higher percentage of residents who were insulin dependent diabetics and many of them had comorbidities associated to their diabetes, such as eye problems, skin and kidney issues. I loved updating and learning how to accommodate these conditions in the aged care setting.

The amount of wound care in a large home was quite a revelation, not because I hadn't encountered it before, but more because of the complexity of the wounds we cared for. We had leg ulcers, cuts and abrasions, aseptic stoma care and even post-operative wound care including suture and clip removal procedures for our convalescent care residents. This was like a blast from the past for me and it reminded me of my time in the hospital setting, but without the NHS pressures. One challenge to the smooth running of these nursing duties was firstly to make sure that we had adequate and appropriate supplies of aseptic supplies like dressing packs, clip removers, suture scissors and wound care products such as adhesive dressings and cleansing solutions. In the nursing home setting, we had to get these items ordered on prescription, then dispensed by the chemist or pharmacy because we had no central store to rely on. Additionally, some medical items had to be sourced from Clacton Hospital surgical supplies. This involved preplanning and holding a small stock for emergencies. I enjoyed preparing wound care treatment charts and plans, working in collaboration with visiting doctors who heavily relied on the qualified nurses for guidance in wound care techniques and treatments as for many of them it had been years since they had last worked in surgery or areas involving wound care. As nurses, we kept ourselves up to date clinically with new products and wound care regimes, partly via the sales representatives that visited nursing homes. They came bearing their goodie bags with samples, cakes and drinks. In exchange we would muster up a group of staff to listen to their pitch and possibly trial the samples, the sales reps hoping that we would then encourage the local doctors to add the product to the resident's prescription.

These sales representatives in the main were ex-qualified nurses and they could very adequately train both nurses and care assistants in stoma care, incontinence aids, mobility equipment, drug use and efficacy, etc. We always looked forward to the Holman representative as he always came laden with a basket of cakes and delicious snacks as a thank you. He wanted us to persuade the management to use their range of incontinence products, on which we spent thousands of pounds, so a few cakes was a worthwhile investment.

The other area of clinical nursing that was in high demand was the use of syringe drivers for end of life, palliative care pain control, something I had only dealt with within the NHS setting. To see, and be responsible for, this in the community was initially daunting, especially on night duty. We used Graseby syringe drivers which administered a precise dose of morphine or other medication evenly over a 24-hour period. The qualified nurse role was to firstly refill the syringe every 24 hours using the controlled drugs protocol and then during that period check it every four hours to ensure that it continued to work according to the prescribed guidelines. We would keep a chart to ensure that the site of the cannula was rotated every 24 hours to a different area.

    I had worked with and used Graseby syringe drivers on Ward 8 at Essex County Hospital at the end of my nurse training and I soon regained my confidence working with them again in the aged care setting. I also had responsibility for ensuring that the junior staff nurses were familiar with both the operation of the syringe drivers and the protocols around their use.

The provision of nurse led tasks, such as the use of syringe drivers for medication purposes, was one of the elements involved in setting the price for a resident's care package, whether they were privately or government funded. The funding of aged care beds was an area in which I had only worked on the periphery of at Seaview and Hill House as I was primarily involved with staffing, training and care provision.

The Carnarvon, as part of a national care home provider group, didn't hide their pricing and all senior staff members who might have encountered prospective residents or their families were given all the information and resources they need to secure a sale. At the time, I intensely disliked the word 'sale' in the nursing home setting, but in real terms that is exactly what it was. There was a variety of funding options for residents and their families. These ranged from means tested local authority funded care packages to partial and fully funded private placements. Now it would be nice to say that all residents were offered the same room options regardless of their funding, but that was not the case. In practice, as in private medicine, if you are fully privately funded you had the options of the best views, single rooms, en-suites and furniture choices, etc., but what all residents, whether local authority or privately funded, had no control over was the staff or the level and standard of care. Everyone was treated the same and I liked that.

I was getting to grips with funding at a time when national and local government aims were to outsource as much as possible to the private sector which helped to support the boom in the private care home business. This outsourcing movement started with the NHS and Community Care Act 1990, which established local authority responsibility for assessing, funding and commissioning care, instead of striving to deliver it in it government owned and run healthcare establishments. This was a welcome development for independent and national care home owners and it also fuelled the need for qualified nurses with ambition to move into senior management within this sector, which had previously been known as 'dead end nursing jobs.' I felt privileged to be part of a change management process that would see increases in single and en-suite rooms for our residents, increased staffing levels and a focus on quality which would be backed up by the care home group striving to achieve the then illustrious ISO 9002, Investors in People award. A mark of quality that helped to keep the fees, the care and service quality standards high.

Chapter Ten: Complex care in nursing homes

One of the big attractions and professional incentives for me, when I was considering the move to a senior role in a large nursing home with a wide variety of residents' conditions catered for, was the opportunity to use my acute care nursing skills outside the hospital environment. Part of the challenge, from a nursing home staffing perspective, was that with a lower percentage of qualified nurse hours available in the aged care setting, it was imperative that as nurses we had the time, equipment and resources to safely deliver and meet the complex care needs of our residents 24 hours a day. So, what complex care skills fell into this category of nurse duties?

Complex care covers a multitude of nursing needs and conditions, but in my experience, some of the most common were peg feeding and care of the gastrostomy site to facilitate enteral feeding, a variety of stomas and their care and tracheostomies. Some of these would already be a challenge to some nurses even in the relative safety of the hospital setting when you had the back up of medical support if problems or complications arose. For example, dealing with a blocked tracheostomy tube in a nursing home requires quick, effective action to be taken backed up by the skill and experience to reassure the residents and endeavour to prevent a reoccurrence. The level of professional responsibility on the nurse in charge was much higher and more critical. To help me explain this in more detail, I have chosen a few complex nursing situations taken from my time working in the nursing home setting and based on my personal experiences:

PEG's and enteral feeding:

PEG stands for Percutaneous Endoscopic Gastrostomy. It is an endoscopic medical procedure (i.e. performed using an **endoscope** which is a long, thin, flexible tube with a light source and camera at one end.) during which a tube is passed into a resident's stomach through the abdominal wall. The PEG insertion procedure does not always require a general anaesthetic, depending on the reason for its insertion. Some long-term PEG's were inserted during major surgery for conditions such as bowel cancer to avoid two procedures.

PEG feeding is used when residents cannot maintain an adequate level of nutrition for health and well-being via their oral intake. The reasons for this can include CVA or strokes causing dysphagia, cancers in oesophagus, throat or bowel causing strictures or obstruction, Crohn's disease or the long-term use of sedation.

Dysphagia is the medical term for difficulty in swallowing. It can be related to certain foods, liquid or consistencies or it can be classified as completed, meaning nothing can be swallowed. Signs and symptoms of dysphagia include choking or coughing whilst eating or drinking, regurgitation of food, via the mouth or through the nose, the sensation of food being stuck in the throat or windpipe or excessive saliva production and dribbling.

The PEG feeding method allows enteral nutrition (which is the provision of nutrients through the gastrointestinal tract when the resident is unable to chew or swallow food, but can digest and absorb nutrients.) This allows the natural digestion process to occur without oral food or fluid consumption. Residents who have suffered a stroke, for example, can have poor or weak swallow reflex muscles and therefore they can be at risk of aspiration pneumonia. (This is an inflammatory condition of the lungs and bronchi caused by inhaling foreign material such as food particles or vomit).

From a nursing perspective, the care of a resident with a PEG feeding regime was focused on ensuring that an adequate supply of the prescribed amount of liquid food was available and administered as ordered. The dietician worked closely with the GP, pharmacy and nursing home staff to ensure there was always the correct amount available for use plus the provision of an adequate supply of the single use tubing sets needed. The monitored dosage pump needed to be well maintained, calibrated and working effectively at all times. The nurse's day to day responsibilities were principally around the administration of the feed, often overnight, with close observation for signs of intolerance, tube blockages or PEG site infection. There were two ways to administer the feed, by pump or by syringe. Syringe feeds were more time intensive because they involved the nurse standing and holding the syringe above the height of the resident and slowly topping it up to allow gravity to administer the feed. Occasionally they were ordered to be slowly pushed in with the plunger but this method increased the risk of vomiting if too much went in too fast. I liked administering by the gravity method as it was an opportunity to chat to the resident, thus distracting them from what was going on and to give them a less clinical feel and approach to this vital process. The syringe administration method usually meant at least three feeds a day just like meals.

Accurate fluid balance charting and stool monitoring for residents undergoing PEG feeding was needed to ensure that their kidneys and bowels were processing the feeds effectively and that they were adequately hydrated. The PEG tubing had to be flushed with 30mls of water before and after each feed to ensure the tube was clear. If the tube became blocked, we would need to try to syringe out the obstruction or try short pressured amounts of water to move the obstruction. Most blockages occurred due to insufficient flushing of the tube after the feed. Enteral feeding solution was very sticky and thicker than milk. If it was spilt would dry to a hard, crusty lump when exposed to air.

Care of the PEG site, usually on the abdomen, was needed daily. With a direct route into the stomach through the abdominal wall, infection of the site needed to be avoided. The other daily checks included making sure the length of the tube, externally, where it goes into the body, was not getting longer or shorter. Too long and it could be leaving the stomach and feed could be entering the abdominal cavity, too short and the tube could be curling up inside and causing resistance during feeding.

After and in between feeds the PEG tube needed to be covered or blocked with a spigot to prevent anything entering or exiting the tube. Residents on enteral feeding were weighed every 3rd day to start with and then weekly once a feeding routine was successfully established.

Stoma care:

In its clinical sense, a stoma can probably best be described as an artificial opening made into a hollow organ, especially on the surface of the body leading to the gut or the trachea. One of the most common stomas we dealt with were colostomies. A colostomy is when a piece of bowel is cut and secured by sutures to an opening in the abdomen so that the content of the bowel's digestive waste can be diverted away from a bowel problem area and collected in a colostomy bag worn over the stoma. The area of the colon being bypassed may have been affected or removed due to cancer or disease. A colostomy can be temporary or permanent. Some of the conditions where a colostomy may be created include injury, bowel cancer, Crohn's disease or diverticulitis

Colostomy residents, particularly the females or younger residents, needed a lot of reassurance and support in addition to the nursing input to help overcome some of the issues that cause personal embarrassment, such as odour control and ensuring the stoma bag is not visible through clothing. Some residents could be taught how to empty the stoma bag and ensure it was properly sealed afterwards to avoid leakage. Care of the stoma site and the changing of the flange that held the bag in place was a nursing task and a good opportunity to check skin integrity near the site as exposure to the acid in digestive waste, infection and skin erosion was a problem if left untreated.

Tracheostomy:

This is a surgical procedure which makes an incision on the front of the neck and creates an opening directly into airway into the trachea or windpipe. The stoma is called a tracheostomy, and it operates as a site for a tracheostomy tube to be inserted and secured by neck tapes. This allows the resident to breath without using their nose or mouth

The reasons for performing a tracheostomy can include tumours, chronic lung conditions, neck or spinal cord issues or trauma. In a nursing home, maintaining the airway via the trachea means that access to suction equipment must be available. A build-up of secretions or blood in the tube can result in death. Therefore, the nursing responsibly is to ensure all staff are observant for signs of obstruction and that nurses and care staff are adequately trained in the use of suction to clear the tube in an emergency. Some relatives of tracheostomy residents were also trained in this.

During 'normal' breathing, our mouth and nose moistens the air and filters debris but when breathing is via a tracheostomy, this doesn't happen and the debris can cause a build up of secretions in the lungs. These secretions often need to be cleared by suctioning through the tracheostomy tube.

In patients with tracheostomies, restricted or total lack of speech is a big challenge. Some residents learn to put their fingers over the tube to allow air to pass through the vocal chords, although there is a risk of infection using this method to communicate. Some other issues faced by tracheostomy residents are reduced appetite and food intake and swallowing problems. If food or secretions enter the lungs it can cause pneumonia or choking.

As you can see in this brief selection of complex care issues, the correct skills and training in the nursing home setting are a vital requirement for all staff involved in the delivery of complex care.

Sarah Jane Butfield

Chapter Eleven: Life at The Carnarvon for our residents

Why are they called residents, and not clients or patients?

This is something often asked by the families of prospective new arrivals and some new members of staff. The term resident didn't seem to equate to the perceived status or needs of the person involved. Initially, when working as a care assistant I thought it was self-explanatory; the person requiring care or supervision was moving to 'reside' in a new home, hence the term resident. However, as the questioning of the term continued I looked deeper into why.

The terminology used to describe the clientele in the various nursing and residential care home facilities that I encountered varied and the words resident, client and patient were the three most common descriptions of the people we cared for.

Resident means: a person who lives somewhere permanently or on a long-term basis.

Client means: a person who pays a professional person or organisation for the provision of a service.

Patient means: a person receiving, or registered to receive, medical treatment. In general, this term is reserved for people receiving care in the hospital, or community, by district nurses or allied health professionals, such as physio or occupational therapists.

The origin of the confusion I think stemmed from the scenarios below:

When someone was being transferred for short stay or respite care they were sometimes referred to 'clients'.

People requiring long term, medically based care, such as end of life/terminal care were frequently referred to as 'patients'.

The long stay, particularly elderly people were called residents. Therefore, in the aged care sector the general term for all service users became residents.

The 60 residents at The Carnarvon were not segregated into mental ability or mobility groups which happened in some homes, the only exception to this being the physical location of the young chronically sick beds when the new wing opened. Our end of life residents, being cared for in single rooms, enabling family and friends to come and go without disturbing the other residents, commanded a higher input of qualified nurse time and attendance, but they were never excluded from the communal events or daily activities.

The mornings were busy in the home, with residents of all abilities being prepared for the first activity of the day, breakfast. They could choose to either sit out at the table in their room or go to the dining room for breakfast. Some residents needed toileting or pressure area care and a full bed bath before being transported to the dining room. In the main, it was our small proportion of residential care residents who managed to shower, wash and dress before breakfast.

The high dependency, principally immobile, residents who had suffered or presented with the after effects of conditions such as strokes (CVA's) as they were known then, chronic breathing impairment conditions such as COPD, or amputation as a consequence of diabetes, etc., often required two-person attention to hoist or manoeuvre them from their beds to bathrooms where they could be prepared for the day. Attention to their personal hygiene needs was given before transferring them by wheelchair or assisting them with mobility aids to the dining room. As a large majority of our high dependency residents required some form of assistance or supervision at meal times, we liked to sit them in the dining room thus allowing a care assistant or nurse to be able to attend to their needs whilst sitting beside them and not standing over them like teachers over a child during an examination which would have been intimidating.

Breakfast is not only a time for eating it is a time for social interaction, the administration of medication and an overall assessment of mood and condition by the qualified nurse in charge. The main medication round took place four times a day and so three of those coincided with meal times. The daily delivery of newspapers that had been requested by residents would arrive in reception and be named by the secretary before distribution by the activities coordinator. The television would be on in the communal areas for much of the day except when entertainment or activities were in progress. It was like a white noise in the background to prevent the stillness of silence which always brought about a sense of solemnness and foreboding. The channel was rarely changed unless a member of staff tried to manipulate the viewing for their own pleasure while attending to residents in the lounge. This was a regular occurrence when long running soaps came on in the evenings, principally EastEnders, Coronation Street and Emmerdale.

As the morning progressed, one by one, the residents appeared in the lounge, either on foot, assisted by Zimmer frames or sticks, or by wheelchair, after washing, showering or bathing. Although I would like to say that personal care and toilet hygiene was not regimented or pre-planned to suit the needs of the home and the staff, to be honest it was. Therefore, the next time orientated task which occurred before lunch was the toileting round. Those residents that were not incontinent were toileted on demand throughout the day. However, the residents with incontinence issues were toileted, had their incontinence pads changed or catheters emptied at prearranged times. The 30 minutes before meals was one of those times. The immobile residents that needed the use of the Arjo or Oxford hoist that we used at The Carnarvon were manoeuvred out of the lounge if possible before being hoisted to preserve some dignity as the placement of the straps between their legs, especially for ladies, was undignified to say the least.

As we had some residents on continuous oxygen therapy the strict enforcement of a 'no smoking' policy was a priority. Despite this, the number of especially pipe smoking residents, and visitors, who seemed to think they were exempt was a problem. One of our COPD residents, who had a portable oxygen therapy unit attached to her wheelchair, which connected to her nose by green, plastic nasal cannula tubing, was always quick to raise the alarm if she saw a pipe being handled, let alone lit. She would yell loudly, "Smoker in the room!" Everyone would turn to look for the culprit.

On a Thursday morning, the mobile hairdresser visited and the residents who had a pre-booked appointment had their hair washed and then they sat near the hairdressing room to wait their turn. For the female residents, in particular, it was a social occasion as they chatted, flicked through magazines and achieved a small slice of normality in an artificial environment.

The stereotypical vision of old people sitting all day in armchairs pushed back against the wall, inhibiting social interaction, was avoided as much as possible by arranging the residents into small groups. However, a few that had hearing or speech impairment seemed to prefer their own company and made a beeline for the solitary chairs and positions when they were available.

With breakfast over and the care assistants busy with the personal hygiene needs of the residents, it was the turn of the cleaning and laundry staff to add to the hustle and bustle of the home. The laundry staff would collect the soiled and used bedding in large sacks on a trolley from the sluices as the care assistants duly filled them as the beds were changed and remade. The turnover of bed linen was continuous and the mornings were focused on that, whereas the afternoon and evening saw the laundering of the residents' personal clothing move to the fore. A wall of coloured, labelled boxes filled the linen room and as the clothes were washed, dried and if necessary ironed they would be placed into the appropriate boxes ready for the night staff to put away into the wardrobes and drawers when they settled the residents into bed.

The never-ending tasks for the cleaners must at times have felt fruitless and unrelenting. As the residents vacated their rooms for the morning the cleaners would open the windows and set about the daily cleaning routines. Despite the continuous cleaning and the welcome fresh sea air, in some areas of the home artificial air fresheners were still needed to disguise the smell of urine. The home was always clean, but the occasional urinary accident or the movement of incontinent residents or wet pads for disposal made distinctive odour unavoidable at times.

Lunchtime arrived and the care assistants gathered at the food hatch, wearing white or blue tabards and waiting for the hot food to arrive. On the first and second floor this was via the dumb waiter, (a small elevator for carrying things, especially food and dishes, between the floors of a building.) There were members of the care team who aspired to a career as nurses and they would regularly ask to assist the nurse on medication duty in preference to feeding or serving at mealtimes.

One of the perceived undignified practices which was aimed at reducing the amount of laundry in the home, already a mammoth undertaking, was the application of washable or disposable bibs to some of the residents at mealtimes. The food was divided into categories depending of the chewing and swallowing capabilities of the residents.

1. Pureed or liquefied for those with poor or impaired swallow reflexes.
2. Mashed or chopped for residents with chewing issues.
3. Normal diet meaning that the only intervention that might be required would be to cut up a piece of meat due to the bluntness of the cutlery.

The practice and skill of feeding was not one that came easily to all staff despite many of them being mums who had spent years feeding their own children as toddlers. I am not sure if it was the fact that they were face to face with an older or obviously disabled person or that they were fearful of them choking but some care assistants needed a lot of support, advice and guidance to enable the experience to become one that both the resident and care assistant could participate in without stress and mess! I know when I had my first experience of feeding a hospital patient during my nurse training I could feel my own mouth opening as I filled the spoon with food and manoeuvred it towards the patient's mouth. This must have looked quite funny to onlookers and I know I was not alone in this involuntary act as I observed it many times in my aged care career when other staff did the same thing.

No matter what the events of the morning had been, after a hearty lunch, a quick look around the lounge would reveal many of our residents catching forty winks (taking a nap) before the afternoon activities commenced.

The television would still be on for those not participating in a snooze as the lounge would be prepared quietly for an afternoon of activity or visiting entertainers. My favourite afternoon visitors were the domestic pets from a local group of animal lovers. It changed each time but there could be a couple of dogs or it could be small pet day with guinea pigs and rabbits. The physical contact with pets brought smiles and induced conversations about pets our residents had cared for or owned in their child or adult life. We had a few ex-farmers and farmer wives, so tales from the farmyard soon took over. On bingo afternoons, the residents would be gathered around the dining table ready to play for prizes which included sweets, books, magazines, etc.

5pm was teatime and usually consisted of soup, sandwiches, salad and cakes. Some residents chose to have this meal in their room as part of their winding down for the day routine so in general we had less residents in the dining room which meant the medication round took a little longer as the trolley would have to do a lap of the home to make sure everyone had their mediation with their meal.

After tea, some of the high dependency residents would start to be returned to their rooms for their night-time preparation routine. This consisted of mouth care, toileting and positioning them into bed by 8pm ready for the final doses of medication for the day and eventually sleep. Part of the holistic approach to the planning of care provision in aged care involved actively working to achieve the wishes of the resident, even in the simplest of things, such as choosing what time to go to bed. Some of them, despite their physical challenges and the tiredness this induced, longed for the time in their room to listen to a favourite radio show like 'The Archers' or watch an episode of their favourite television show, without the melee of the nursing home routines interrupting them. It wasn't always possible to achieve this, but we tried.

It's night time and with the arrival of the night staff a couple of hours of intense activity occurs, but without excess noise or disruption.

The remaining residents are returned to their rooms and settled into bed. Call bells are answered for residents requiring toileting, something to drink or to reassure them if they are confused as the night time approaches. The qualified nurse on duty makes her rounds checking the residents and administering the night time medication. The highlight for some residents at this time of day is the arrival of the hot drinks trolley as the care assistant arrives with insulated jugs filled with hot chocolate, Horlicks, warm milk or any other hot drink requested. The residents who require assistance with their hot drinks are attended to last to ensure they are not rushed. On night duty, the background noise in the home, before everyone is asleep, consists of a mixture of sounds from radio and television programmes penetrating the doors of the resident's rooms due to the volume some of them needed it at. This was occasionally interrupted by a confused resident calling out, or the sound of the nurse call system before it is put onto night mode with a quieter tone. The residents would be attended to on demand or checked hourly during the night by the nursing and care staff discreetly to avoid waking them or the other residents unnecessarily.

Sarah Jane Butfield

Chapter Twelve: Perception versus reality of being an aged care nurse

There was, and still is, in some places, a harsh perception that the qualified nurses who work in aged care do so because they 'are not good enough or can't get a job in a hospital' or that they are approaching retirement and want an 'easy job'. Aged care nursing is not an easy job, by any stretch of the imagination, if it is performed well and in the pursuit of high standards of care provision. If anything, the medical assessment skills and ability to deal efficiently with medical and emergency situations by nurses in some aged care settings means that they are more highly skilled in some aspects of skill assessments than some hospital based nurses. In addition, because of this requirement in their role, many aged care nurses adamantly pursue their professional development and ongoing education ensuring that they are above the average or mandatory requirements to maintain their registration.

The nurse recruitment crisis that exists today in aged care is clearly linked to pay, but when I worked in aged care the pay rates were more than comparable, and for senior nurses often exceeded NHS pay rates, as did the work life balance incentives, such as flexi-time and split shifts. Today, nursing and care homes find it hard to recruit nurses and recruit heavily from overseas.

There is an increasing reliance on agency nurses meaning that homes cannot always provide the continuity of care which is vital in the nursing home setting. Nurses need to know their residents and their capabilities to accurately identify their individual care needs and spot deterioration or medical issues that require intervention and treatment.

In the 1990s however there were plenty of benefits to working in a nursing home for qualified nurses. The nursing environment and ethos of care evoked and encouraged a real sense of team work, which in turn led to the levels of job satisfaction being higher. As an example, the care planning and implementation of nursing processes involved with nursing residents with dementia, Alzheimer's, and an array of mental health conditions was extremely rewarding. The pursuit of ensuring that the residents achieved a good quality of life was extremely fulfilling and heart-warming.

Being able to spend a substantial amount of time working hands-on with the care assistants and the residents meant that the nursing staff were on top of any changes in the resident's skin condition, breathing, dietary intake, etc., much quicker than they would have been if they were working in the acute sector. The myths that nurses in aged care don't acquire, need or retain their clinical skills was in my experience completely unfounded.

I would go as far as to say that given the acute care nursing tasks I handled daily in the aged care setting which included colostomies, urostomies, ileostomies, urinary catheters, tracheostomies, enteral feeding, etc., my skillset and knowledge base expanded extensively. In addition, in aged care, a resident's physical condition can worsen rapidly and nurses need to be able to communicate precisely and succinctly with the on-call doctors, receptionists and paramedics to facilitate the most timely and appropriate emergency treatment, attendance or action required.

Nursing shifts were on average eight to ten hours during the days and twelve hours at night. Almost fifty percent of that could be filled with the administration, and ordering of medications. Other daily tasks included wound care, liaising with GPs, other members of the allied health care team, formulating and updating care plans and completing patient centred risk assessments. These included moving and handling, infection control, skin integrity, etc. The ongoing daily shift management of the care assistants to ensure that the appropriate resident allocation was made, based on the care needs of the residents and skills available from the staff on duty, was a careful balancing act, with tact, diplomacy and often conflict management skills required! Working hands on also gave the qualified nurse team the opportunity to immediately address training needs and concerns in real time rather than having to schedule a meeting or training session when the initial reason for the training may well have been forgotten, or no longer existed.

Aged care qualified nurses played a key role in developing the skills and knowledge of the care assistants many of whom started with little or no experience. Even among the 'experienced care assistants' regular assessment of their skills was needed to ensure best practice was implemented at all times.

It was commonplace for impromptu daily training sessions to occur on subjects ranging from infection control to feeding techniques. Being a nurse in a nursing home can be every bit as busy, frustrating and rewarding as working in any other healthcare environment. I liked going to work and seeing the same residents every shift. Looking back with pride in my professional career fulfilment, I can hand on heart say that my years in aged care enhanced my career, increased my skill set and gave me immense job satisfaction. I adored working with the elderly and I thrived on the challenge of caring for our young chronically sick residents in what many of them perceived as an alien, sometimes socially unacceptable, setting.

What professions form part of the allied healthcare teams that support aged care services and what do nurses gain from working alongside them?

Here are some of the professionals that I came into contact with during my aged care career:

Art Therapist

Music Therapist

Chiropodist

Podiatrist

Dietitian

Hearing aid dispenser

Occupational Therapist

Paramedic

Physiotherapist

Counselling psychologist

Prosthetist

Radiographer

Social worker

Speech and Language Therapist

As you can see they cover a diverse range of healthcare needs, but all play an integral part in providing holistic, resident centred care packages. The abilities, disabilities or impairment of the individual resident forms part of a nurse or doctor's assessment of the additional allied healthcare input required. As many nursing home residents have some form of funding assistance or funding advice before admission, most have already been assessed or had input from the social work team, either in the hospital setting or at home. Social workers play a big part in helping residents and their families make the right choice when finding a nursing home placement, alongside helping them to organise and manage the financial and social based aspects that a move to an aged care facility brings.

In relation to a resident's physical well-being, and the provision of their ongoing healthcare needs, let us take, for example, an elderly person who has suffered a stroke. They may suffer from some form of physical disability in the form of paralysis or weakness in limbs, which can result in limited or impaired mobility, and a tendency for spasms or contracted limbs. The advice and support of the physiotherapist is crucial to achieve maximum restoration of limb use and establish ongoing management once the limit of recovery has been achieved. They are also responsible for the assessment, prescription and use of mobility, lifting and transfer aids such as Zimmer frames, tripod walking sticks, hoist and slide boards. Nurses in aged care are responsible for the implementation of physiotherapy plans and the day to day assessment of needs. The active and passive exercise programs that are documented for the nursing home staff to use are specific to each resident, and their individual pieces of equipment would sometimes involve the physiotherapist providing training to a core group of nursing home staff so that they could roll out the training to their peers.

The input by dieticians is crucial for many nursing home residents, whether it is to accommodate physical impairment in the eating and swallowing mechanics, such as dysphagia, (difficulty with swallowing,) or to ensure adequate nutrition is achieved in residents for whom the act of eating and drinking causes distress. An example of this was dementia residents who needed feeding due to concentration and attention span issues and who forgot to chew properly and were therefore a choking risk. Dieticians would leave detailed instructions for the chef and the nursing and care staff on food consistency, frequency and feeding set up protocols such as the physical positioning of the residents and the feeding aids required and so on.

Communication with residents is vital even if they are deemed to be self caring in other areas. The passing of information to the residents for health, safety and well-being comes down to speech, hearing and sight. If any of these are impaired, then communication and understanding can be affected. A key role for nursing staff is to ensure that residents are regularly assessed for sensory impairment or difficulties and that referrals are made to the appropriate allied healthcare team members for assessment to take place. This process enables the necessary aids to be prescribed and provided to enhance the sensory abilities of the residents. Speech can be impaired through trauma or strokes and the speech therapist often works hand in hand with the dietician especially in the treatment and management of dysphagia.

These examples demonstrate the importance and relevance of a team focused approach to aged care and the individual requirements of the residents being cared for. The complex and varied range of medical conditions, disabilities and nursing care needs within the aged care sector makes the partnership between the allied healthcare team and the home managers and nursing teams vital. An abundance of knowledge, expertise and experience was available, shared and information gleaned for future reference and use and for me personally this aspect of holistic care planning would come to the fore again in my career in a few years' time.

Sarah Jane Butfield

Chapter Thirteen: Upskilling and discovery!

Within a couple weeks of my starting work at The Carnarvon in March 1993 the home manager, Annette, had started to discuss the possibly of training me up to cover for her as 'temporary Home Manager' as she had some long overdue annual leave to book. The other senior sisters were not interested in providing her holiday cover or accepting the increased temporary responsibility, but I revelled in the opportunity to learn how the management role differed as part of a national care home group from that of a privately-owned nursing home.

When the time came for my secondment into the four-week temporary position as home manager I was mentored by Area Manager, Liz Jennings and the Regional Manager, Tony Barrow. They oozed knowledge, experience and expertise and like a sponge I stayed close and attentive to absorb it. During this period, I worked Monday to Friday 8.30am – 5pm. My new duties and responsibilities included daily checks on the residents, I liked to do this at breakfast time in case I spotted anyone who should be added to the visiting doctor's list for the day. There was an array of daily correspondence to read, action and file appropriately. The follow up of any outstanding new residents' enquiries needed constant attention to keep our respite and convalescence beds full. I dealt with head office enquiries in relation to all aspects of the home's running including operational and financial matters, in addition to ensuring that staffing levels were maintained and that any sickness absences were covered immediately, whether it was nursing, care, kitchen or cleaning staff. However, one of my primary roles was to be the 'go to' person for the nursing staff for any discussions, advice or support with decisions on medical or care provision matters.

This experience was an interesting and educational introduction into how a national care home operates from the boardroom down to local nursing and residential home level. It gave me a valuable insight that, when my secondment was complete, helped me to appreciate and identify areas of opportunity within the qualified nurse role for making changes that would ultimately result in a higher standard of care provision for our residents. It also enabled me to think outside the box in relation to staff friendly methods of working to improve morale and education in basic care provision skills. I was so inspired by the experience that I used any spare time that I had compiling a summary of my thoughts, observations and ideas for ways to improve. Upon reflection, I must have appeared overzealous and possibly perceived by Annette as a threat. Either that or I was being critical of her management techniques, but that was never my intention. I wanted to work with her from the nursing and care side of the home's operation to give her help and support. Initially, she brushed off my ideas and I knew her copy of my ideas lay unread on top of the filing cabinet as I saw it there every day that I was on shift as I collected the drug cupboard keys. It slowly became obscured with items being placed on top of it. The lack of interest soon dampened my enthusiasm and I settled back into my nursing role determined to find enjoyment in the clinical side of things for myself and our residents. I was still responsible for training the care assistants and I even interviewed potential new ones when Annette was double booked or unavailable, as we needed not only a core of staff, but also a large bank of casual staff for holiday, sick and maternity leave. Therefore, we never passed up the opportunity to interview someone with experience and/or a good-looking CV.

From a personal perspective, life had improved dramatically and Jack was presenting himself as the attentive partner and started to properly bond with the children, Robert in particular. I don't recall what triggered it, whether it was the loss of my mum or the strength of Jack's desire to become a dad but we agreed to try for a baby and I was pregnant within a month of stopping my contraceptive pill. It was hard to get excited in the early weeks of the pregnancy, after the trauma of my miscarriage previously, but when I reached 20 weeks a sense of relief set in and I could really enjoy being pregnant. Annette, the staff and residents were all thrilled for me and as I ballooned in size and trundled around in my white starched maternity uniform dress, which made me resemble a walking tent, I truly believed I had made it through more than enough tough personal times, but that now aged 28 I had finally sorted myself and my career out. I worked up to 33 weeks then started my maternity leave.

As we excitedly prepared for the birth, pre-eclampsia stuck again and I was admitted to hospital. Jack was taking sole care of Samantha and Robert with the support of his mother and as they had school during the day as well I had no obvious concerns. Samantha was 7 and Robert 5 and they too were looking forward to a little brother or sister. After being induced at just under 37 weeks I gave birth to our beautiful baby girl Molly May in February 1994. I remember this being the only moment, in our long and turbulent relationship, that Jack kissed me on the head, as the midwife was wrapping Molly up to hand to me. He told me he loved me and I believed he meant it.

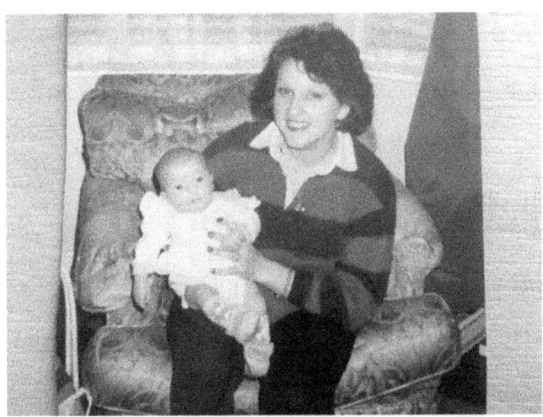

Sarah Jane and Molly

Our little family settled into new routine quickly and the days and weeks flew by and when Jack proposed to me in March there seemed no reason to say no. We were married in April 1994. A few close friends commented on how quickly it happened, but Jack arranged it all. I didn't think anything of it at the time, but clearly, I should have, because within two weeks of being married Jack and Molly were gone!

It took a few days to locate and contact him and even then I got little information on why and what had happened to cause this traumatic separation. Jack was adamant that he was doing what was best for him and Molly and I am not sure if it was the fact that I was still in the early months of the post-natal period, but I felt as if my body and mind wanted to shut down. I knew I had to fight for Molly because I truly believed she should be with her mum and her siblings. I believed we should all be together, I thought he loved us all. Our relationship deteriorated as the battle commenced and my physical condition followed. I was diagnosed with post-natal depression but the antidepressant therapy and counselling did nothing to relieve the pain in my heart as I remained separated from my baby.

Over the years that I had been in a 'relationship' with Jack I had learned a few things that sometimes worked to draw him back into the relationship but this time my desperation for Molly seemed to push him further away. I knew that I could not fight this battle alone and reluctantly I consulted a family law specialist. I had no idea at that time that the key to Jack's success in keeping me from my beautiful baby daughter was the fact that we had married and he now legally had shared parental responsibility. Was the wedding a ploy to achieve this horrific end game result? I still like to think not, but I am long past thinking I know anything about the workings of his mind. The legal wrangling was going to be expensive and I didn't qualify for legal aid as I was technically full time employed even though my maternity leave would be ending soon and I would need to return to work.

The solicitor I was consulting was very clear that I must maintain contact with jack at all costs to enable us to know where they were and to be able to review whether he was indeed taking good care of Molly. I had no doubts on that. He loved her, and over the weeks and months after he left, when I did get a brief visit or meeting with my daughter, she always had designer clothes and the very best baby equipment in tow. I tried to let my family in to support me but I felt ashamed at having been fooled again and I felt everyone observing this disastrous situation was judging me. I appreciate now that it must have looked from the outside that I had just let her go, but that was so far from the truth. I dare not explain the lengths I went to so that I could be rewarded with a few hours with my baby or sometimes even an overnight stay.

Now the harsh reality of the financial cost was setting in as the legal bills mounted as did the debt from our joint accounts, which had been maxed out in the period after he left. I had to return to work as soon as possible to try and resolve this, but worse still I now faced the prospect of losing the home which I had intended to provide financial security and a settled home for Samantha and Robert. I returned to work and over the next few months I tried to start chipping away at the debt but it was futile. A more effective course of action was needed. I needed a miracle. I hoped and prayed that one day I would be forgiven for my weakness of mind, naivety and ignorance. Everyone around me at work tried to support me, and I was fortunate to make a good friend called Lynnette who was a newly qualified Registered Nurse at The Carnarvon. Although she was young, newly qualified and not a mum herself, this did not prevent her being able to be objective, forthright and brutally honest when the need arose. I cried a lot, and tried to do it in private. I had a professional role to fulfil and I needed to maintain my dignity and the professional respect of the staff in my workplace. However, one day after one of my distressed meltdowns in the staffroom, thinking I was alone, a voice startled me.

"Look at yourself Sarah, you are a mess. Is this how you want your kids to remember their mum?"

It was Lynnette. Those words resonated, within me as immediately images of my late mum flooded my mind. Although my childhood had not been perfect or entirely conventional, the one thing that was maintained throughout was the love of my mum. She was always there to pick me up when I fell, hug me when I was hurt and she provided for me and my sisters as a single mum without ever showing us her personal pain. We didn't see any of that until we started to approach adulthood and started to acknowledge and realise the struggles and battles she had fought for us girls. Now look at me. What would my children remember about their childhood? A mum who let a man ruin her life, steal their siblings and almost destroy her making their mum into a sad, woman with no self-esteem acting like a victim and operating from the shell of the person she used to be.

Lynnette was right, I didn't want my kids to remember me like that and I had to do something to change even just my superficial appearance whilst I sorted out life for me and the children.

Chapter Fourteen: Practicalities of independence

Being in the throes of a toxic relationship and not knowing how to escape it in addition to not having the mental strength or courage to cut Jack out without losing contact with Molly meant that I had to act in other ways to secure some form of independence and make myself believe that I did not deserve to be treated this way. Jack became increasingly distant and my contact with Molly became erratic as he entered a new relationship with a woman with two children of a similar age. They set up as the new family unit and there was no place for me without a fight. However, I sensed that he was not going to let me go completely and he used Molly as the tool to achieve that this time. Over the next few months I focused on spending quality time with my children, mum, sisters and my work and my life improved. I started to take positive action to resolve my financial problems and we moved to a small rented ground floor flat in Clacton near the railway station, in walking distance from the seafront, which was great for me and the children, and I could walk to work.

Two new chapters in my life started to happen over the next few weeks and I did believe that my prayers were being answered, although Lynnette told me in no uncertain terms that I had made it happen and that I needed to believe in myself instead of a higher power!

Firstly, I decided that if I could learn to drive then myself and my children would have more freedom and opportunities available to us. I had my provisional licence so all I needed was the lessons. I had the time now as I was living in Clacton surrounded by willing friends who would sit with Samantha and Robert. All I needed was the passion and, of course, the skills. The second event was that Annette resigned from the role of home manager, with immediate effect, for family reasons. The regional manager, Tony, asked me to step in as acting home manager and invited me to apply for the permanent position. I thought initially that I was in no way mentally ready for that kind of interview or application process, although I knew I could handle the acting role. However, as I stepped into the temporary home manager role again to cover during the recruitment process, I regained my sense of professional self-worth again and I sailed through the series of interviews and testing. I was appointed to the role of home manager with a very generous salary and annual leave entitlement, great working hours and working conditions. Suddenly the clouds started to lift from my life and a ray of sunshine appeared.

Taking driving lessons proved to be a bit more dramatic. To be honest, driving did not come naturally. At the time, I thought this was because in my young adult years, people who wanted to learn to drive did so as soon as they left school or college. They did this at a time when their brains were geared up to learning new practical skills. I had no need or desire to learn to drive at that time and so now in my late twenties, I felt like an old woman when I swapped over with a lanky teenager at the start of my lesson. My lessons initially took place in Clacton, but as I progressed I ventured into Colchester and that was a culture shock after the relative quiet of the roads in a seaside town. Despite this I pushed on, but not without having to change my instructor mid-way due to an incident during a lesson, when he shouted at me without explanation. Looking back, I think my fragile emotional condition led me to overreact instead of retaliating. So I did the text book mirror, signal, manoeuvre and pulled the car safely to a stop at the side of the road and got out. Standing on the grass verge, he swore at me instead of trying to find out why I had taken this course of action. He demanded that I get back in, but I was too afraid now. I refused, so he threw my bag out of the window and drove off. I never saw or heard from him again. I found a new instructor and immediately realised I had been hindered by my predecessor and within a few weeks I had put in for my driving test. I passed first time and although I didn't have a car of my own I was excited to share the news.

The ANS head office management team sent me a card to congratulate me on adding this new and valuable skill to my CV and the following week, when Liz and Tony visited from head office to go through the monthly variance accounts, Liz presented me with the keys to a company car, a red Vauxhall Astra estate. I did wonder why they came in two cars that day instead of one! The independence I sought was now a reality, if I was brave enough to take it. With my newly acquired resources in my quest for independence, my beautiful children and I had the opportunity to make a new secure future for ourselves and possibly have some awesome adventures.

It is strange how emotionally strong achieving something, that most might take for granted, made me feel and it induced a spark of hope for the future. I knew that I had the chance to start to break free, and knowing that I could take the children anywhere, anytime was exhilarating. I started driving to Ipswich to visit my sisters more often and the strength of mind and improved focus on what I wanted to achieve in life increased with each dose of inspirational advice I accepted.

On her next visit to the home, Liz asked if I would be willing to join a multidisciplinary team of internal auditors. She explained that as I was the youngest and the newest home manager, I would make a valuable addition to the team. This team would form part of the process of implementation of ISO 9002 and the potential achievement of the IIP - Investors in People Award. Of course, I agreed as I was excited to be part of a new project and to be involved from day one, in addition to the fact that it was uncharted territory for me. The more I read about it, the more the benefits to the residents, staff and the company became apparent.

I had to complete a formal application to attend the internal audit training course in a few weeks time. My application was successful and I then had to work to find someone to cover me when I was sent to Meadbank in London to attend the training and to take part in the first meeting of the new ISO/IIP Team.

So what is ISO 9002 in relation to nursing and residential homes?

ISO 9002 is part of a set of standards in the ISO 9000 group, often referred to as QMS quality management systems, aimed at helping care homes ensure, and prove, that they strive to fully meet the needs of the residents, staff and other 'stakeholders', in addition to meeting statutory and regulatory requirements related to their service provision. Basically, what we were implementing was a system of accountability that, during its implementation, would ensure every aspect of the service we provided would be documented, tried and tested and that internal checks would be put in place to ensure that the service was consistently at a high standard.

To put this in context and to demonstrate the origin of ISO some of you may have been familiar or have heard of BSI, the British Standards Institution also a quality checking and implementation process of assessment and awarding of achievement.

We were implementing the 1987 Model for QA (Quality Assurance).

Focusing on development, implementation, monitoring and best practice service provision, but making our primary focus on the 1994 update which was geared towards preventative measures. That meant we didn't just focus on the end point service delivery but also implemented QA systems to improve the content of the services, identify potential issues and challenges to enable preventative measures to be triggered and actions to be taken.

Each organisation that implemented the QA process was assessed by an independent third party to ensure that all the requirements of the ISO process were met and demonstrated as being adhered to.

The quality management systems we worked on were based on eight key principles which formed the foundations of the standards we were introducing and which would be assessed:

1 – Focus on the Residents

Care home groups depend on their residents and local authority that fund the outsourcing of care therefore it is imperative that as an organisation managers understand current and future service provision needs and plan to meet all the regulatory requirements and strive to exceed service delivery expectations.

2 – Focus on Leadership

Leaders must be able to create and maintain the internal structure and workforce resources to enable staff at all levels to become fully involved in achieving the organisation's objectives and they should do this by establishing a sense of purpose and direction.

3 – Focus on People

People at every stage and in every part of the homes operation are the lifeblood of the group and their total commitment and involvement enables their valuable skills and experience to be shared for the benefit of the residents, staff and the home.

4 – Focus on Processes

Each process, new or existing must be evaluated to ensure that the anticipated result is achieved, with the efficient use of people and resources monitored and managed as a part of a process.

5 – Focus on Management

Best practice in management must involve identifying, understanding and connecting processes to form a system of working that results in effective and efficient achievement of the homes mission statement and its objectives.

6 – Focus on Continual Growth & Improvement

Continual growth and improvement of people and resources must be ongoing, planned, monitored and maintained.

7 – Focus on Decision Making

Decision making at all levels must be based on facts and evidence based data to ensure effective decisions are made and can be proven.

8 – Focus on Professional Relationships

Professional relationships, both internally and externally with the home's suppliers, enable the focus to be on providing high quality service provision, which ultimately creates value for the group and end service users, i.e. our residents.

The formation of the multidisciplinary team, together with the huge time and resources investment needed to make good sound financial business sense. So what did ANS hope to achieve by making this investment? We aimed to attain a high reputation and an increase in new business achieved by offering the highest proven standards of service provision. We did it, and The Carnarvon was awarded the Investors in People Award. The logo was proudly added to all our stationery, literature and merchandise with the Award plaque clearly on display. For years after I left this was maintained. However, I have discovered while connecting with friends in Clacton during my research for this book, that after the home was acquired by another large care home group the standards were not maintained and the home is being considered for closure. If that happens it will be a sad end to a prestigious nursing home.

Chapter Fifteen: A new wing opens!

Due to the age and origins of the main building there had been extensive internal structural changes already during the conversion of The Carnarvon into a nursing home, for example corridor and door widening, the adding of en-suites, etc. Despite this ANS decided to invest further, with the addition of a dedicated wing within the home, suitable and equipped for the provision of high quality, complex care to the young chronically sick, long and short stay residents. The aim of the new wing was to provide age appropriate resources for their physical and psychological care needs. From the physical perspective, it would allow access to the large, sometimes more specialised equipment utilised by this group of residents, including mobility aids, battery powered scooters, hoists, PEG (Percutaneous endoscopic gastrostomy) enteral nutrition and feeding machines, etc.

The investment by the company would provide 15 dedicated rooms; 10 long stay and 5 for respite care packages. The new layout and additional facilities included an adapted kitchenette to allow independence for the making of drinks and snacks, which also allowed residents to entertain their family and friends. A visitor lounge area and a large shower room with high and low wash basins were also included. In addition, the bedrooms had electric and battery powered Kings Fund beds, high-low chairs and new hoists with specialised slings, with controls which some residents would be able to use for themselves to further increase independence with movement and transferring. One of the post important new aspects of this wing was the decoration. The aim was to make it feel distinctly different to the rest of the home and allow long stay residents to individualise their rooms. New bedding, carpets, colour schemes were introduced and these younger residents were able to have items from home with them.

The plans had already been drawn up, approved and the time frames set, before I took the reins as home manager. Therefore, my role was to oversee the building work, in collaboration with the area manager, to coordinate the internal finishing, to plan, organise and host the launch, but most importantly to ensure it would achieve full occupancy within four weeks of opening. The importance of achieving full occupancy of the new wing was drilled into me at every management meeting during the building process. In addition, any residents' rooms that would become vacant in the main nursing home due to transfers to the YCS wing needed to be booked for occupation again as soon as possible. My aims and objectives centred around ensuring that the whole process caused minimal disruption to existing residents and the staff caring for them. However, the distraction of the numerous tanned, muscular building labourers was difficult for some staff and a few cheeky female residents to resist. There was a marked increase in the amount of makeup being worn by our female staff and a few of our young, female care assistants found the distraction of tee-shirt clad, sometimes topless, builders too much to ignore! Even the kitchen assistants tried getting in on the act by volunteering days in advance to do the tea rounds for the workers. The amount of time some staff members spent in the building at the end of their shifts was amusing, as were the excuses they made for being there! Maintaining a safe working and living environment when building works were being carried out, whether internally or externally, was quite a feat at times.

From a business management prospective, I enjoyed working on the capital expenditure budget and implementing the sourcing of the new equipment, furnishings and planning for the redecoration. Each month I would painstakingly compile the reports and figures to demonstrate that we were on course and of course on budget. After all, from the company perspective, I was new to the organisation and in hindsight they had placed a great deal of faith and trust in someone so young.

I devised an assessment tool for the existing young chronically sick residents, to establish if they would be suitable or interested in transferring the new wing. It was by no means a foregone conclusion that they wanted to move, as many were very settled in their rooms and routines and did not relish the chance that anything would be changed to the detriment of the level of contentment and care they received within the home. Working closely with the local healthcare professionals I soon had a short list of potential new residents to follow up with and I was confident of achieving the targets in the business plan. The next objective was to meet the increased staffing and logistical requirements that an extra 15 beds would make. There were many meetings with the senior sisters and other qualified nurses, group meetings of the combined nursing and care team and independent meetings with the kitchen and laundry and maintenance staff. An increase in residents would affect every aspect of the home from meals to laundry; medication to activities, and no element of the residents' or staff's daily routine could be overlooked. It was for this reason that we also had to address the need for a part time assistant for the activities coordinator, especially, if we were to achieve our claims of offering age appropriate entertainment, cultural and pastoral care and individualised support.

As I alluded to earlier chapters, there were some additional and enhanced challenges that needed to be addressed and overcome as part of the package of caring for and accommodating residents in this category and age group.

These included:

The emotional and social stigma of living or receiving respite care in a building clearly called a nursing home and where many of the residents were aged over 60. Would a young person want to encourage friends to come and visit them there? Would they prefer to shut themselves off from the local community and would this lead to isolation and impact their mental well-being?

The psychological issues of acceptance, anger, resentment. Some of these would be aimed at family members who had reached the painful decision that they were unable to cope with the care needs in the home environment, thus leading to the need for a nursing home placement. Many YCS residents struggled with acceptance of their condition particularly if they had an able-bodied life before the development of a lifelong injury or illness.

Many YCS residents who had their disability, disease or any form of physical or psychological impairment since birth had, most of the time already reached some degree of acceptance and their anger, if it presented, was more focused on the frustration of losing certain aspects of their independence.

The need for ongoing access to rehabilitation services, to maintain health and promote independence was a key feature, and our ability to work closely with rehabilitation professionals helped to ensure that we were addressing as many of the potential challenges that this group of residents faced and needed to deal with on a daily basis.

Maintaining a social connection with their age peer group meant that they needed access to places, resources and events that able-bodied adults had. This is where the additional help for the provision of activities, both within the home and attendance at external events, was crucial. The absence of meaningful connections and access to their family, friends and local community could have a huge impact on the approach they took to life and their condition.

Many of their physical care needs were more complex than those of the elderly, due to their age, their conditions and the expected deterioration, particularly in diseases such as Huntington's Disease or MS. When they know that certain abilities will become impaired as the disease progresses this can induce depression related to what lies ahead including further loss of independence.

The training of nursing home staff to be able to deliver the basic personal care required, in a manner that addressed the psychological challenges faced by such residents was a challenge to begin with. Although we already had a small number of YCS residents, the ethos of the new wing was that we were providing specialist care and services which meant that the knowledge and skills of the nursing and care team needed to be fit for purpose. It was not enough that they knew how to provide personal care. For example, there was a need to train staff to recognise and report the early signs of anxiety and depression, when their skills to date had been primarily geared to the delivery of personal hygiene. This training involved the use of workshops, role play and the support of the allied healthcare team.

As the building works progressed we aimed to have two rooms ready ahead of the launch. We wanted these as showrooms to enable viewing by potential residents and their families, but also to demonstrate the facilities to local healthcare professionals, doctors, social workers, rehabilitation consultants, etc., who would hopefully consider referring residents to us. To make good use of these two showrooms, we held two separate open house events. The first was for healthcare professionals, inviting them to come and view the rooms, look at the plans for the new services and facilities and to find out more about the services we offered, and intended to offer. We also encouraged them to make suggestions on equipment, resources, etc., in the hope that this would result in them recommending or referring residents to us.

We answered questions about how the new wing would integrate into the existing nursing home operation and the benefits of this new service to the local community. The staff who were now fully trained in this new category of residents demonstrated equipment and answered questions about their training and professional development. All of this was backed up by our Investors in People work that was going on in the background.

The second event was to promote the new wing and proposed new service to prospective residents and their families. We held an open afternoon with a display featuring the activities and events and age appropriate resources which we were making available.

The main event would be the grand opening and it was my job to find a local or national celebrity to cut the ribbon and hopefully attract some media attention. As this was a seaside town with two established theatres which had summer shows running I decided to approach the theatres to see if any of the acts, which included singers, comedians, actors and musicians could oblige.

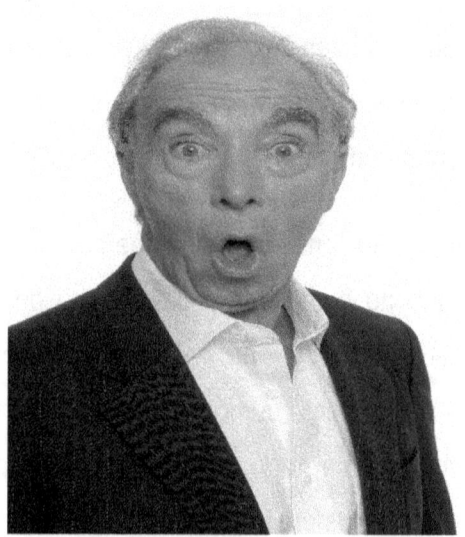

Bernie Clifton

(Image supplied by, and used with the permission of, Greg Day, Clout Communications on behalf of Bernie Clifton)

Our invitation was eventually accepted by a comedian and television presenter, Bernie Clifton, real name Bernie Quinn.

He started out as a singer in pubs and clubs around Blackpool before finding fame as television presenter Crackerjack. In the entertainment world, he was best known for his comedy act involving Oswald the ostrich.

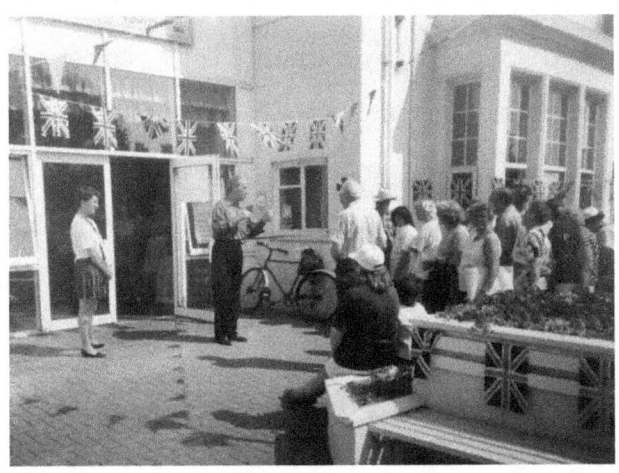

Sarah Jane watches as Bernie Clifton opens the new wing at The Carnarvon

The grand opening and launch day was a huge success. On a hot summers day, we had entertainers, a bouncy castle, food and craft stalls, balloons and of course plenty of internal and external bunting. At the time the Carnarvon was a prestigious home, with an excellent reputation and an established, successful nursing home business. This new venture was a further feather in the ANS cap, but on a local level it made The Carnarvon the home of choice for many, thus our waiting list for both YCS and aged care placements grew.

On a personal note the evening's entertainment and events, which was for the staff, builders, decorators and contractors only, as a thank you, was the first time I had socialised in a very long time. Although I was content as a working, single mum to Samantha and Robert, I still struggled with only part time access to my beautiful baby girl Molly. I had no desire to seek out or enter another relationship in hurry, but this was a rare occasion when one of our local tradesmen started to obviously flirt with me and it felt nice. It made me wonder if I would ever find love or happiness again or if the manipulative hold Jack had over me with Molly truly had ruined any chance of future happiness.

Chapter Sixteen: Let us entertain you

A large part of the home manager role was to maintain full occupancy of the beds in the home, of which there were now 60, and to support this with a waiting list to ensure a profitable income flow. A variety of methods were employed. Some were national initiatives and company led and some were locally led and managed solely by the home manager. A key feature of the offering to residents within an ANS home was the appointment of a full-time Activities Coordinator. This position was perceived by some as a luxury and hence became a low priority in some small, privately owned homes. However, ANS homes, which in the main had a higher number of residents knew and appreciated the value of the role in attracting and retaining residents, making it a worthwhile and lucrative investment.

We had a creative, caring and compassionate activities coordinator during my time at The Carnarvon. Kim, formerly a care assistant, was a chatty, people loving person and we became good friends, since the home manager and the activities coordinator worked very closely together on a variety of projects and duties. The role was not solely centred on providing entertainment for the residents, but it also played a key role in supporting the nursing and care staff in the social, emotional and pastoral care needs of our residents. That's not to say that we didn't incorporate some of the stereotypical nursing home pastimes such as bingo and dominoes!

Kim organised the newspapers order with the secretary each morning just like in a hotel. She coordinated appointments with the mobile hairdresser, who visited every Thursday, and appointments for the monthly chiropodist visit in liaison with the qualified nurses. She provided a vital support service as well as being a good listener and taking time to chat to and listen to the residents on a one to one basis. They would often confide their medical and social problems to her enabling her to facilitate access to solutions.

The home had a rolling program of events which would be pre-planned to enable staffing, transport and funding to be secured well in advance. The activities and events included a monthly visiting marketplace where outside contractors would come in with clothes, gifts, and crafts to sell. This was popular with the more immobile residents who were less likely to come with us on the external shopping excursions by minibus to nearby towns. They enjoyed having the opportunity to choose and buy birthday and Christmas cards and gifts for family and friends, giving them a much need slice of independence.

We would also take groups of residents out each month on trips to the Prince's Theatre in Station Road, Clacton. The support team would consist of me, Kim and some volunteer care assistants who were rewarded with a ticket to watch the show for free in return for helping to push wheelchairs to the theatre or help with residents on the minibus if we had a larger group. We watched everything from ballet to pantomime, movies to poetry recitals. I became quite cultured for a while. A highlight for me was when we took ten residents to a screening of Four Weddings and Funeral, one of my all-time favourite films which I have watched probably over 20 times. One of the stars of the show was Scottish actress Elspet Gray, wife of Lord Rix, who was in Clacton for the screening. She played the mother of the bride in the first wedding. When the content of the show was age appropriate I would buy tickets so that Samantha and Robert could attend as well. Samantha was like a miniature care assistant straightening residents lap blankets and checking if they needed a drink, a tissue or popcorn! As we sometimes had a large group booking we would, on selected occasions, be offered the chance to meet the cast members with the residents after the show. The residents loved this, it made them, 'feel like royalty' as one resident used to say.

Kim and I acquired a nickname for one of our more solemn, yet responsible roles, which that was important for the residents, the staff and the home's reputation. We were the 'professional funeral goers'. We attended all funerals of residents who died whether they were in the home or in hospital at the time. From a company and professional standpoint, it was a mark of respect and we represented the home, the staff the other residents' and ANS. In a personal capacity, some of the residents were like family to us, each with their own personalities and individual traits. Bereavement in the aged care setting must be sensitively handled with respect for the deceased their family and friends but also recognising and taking into consideration the relationships and friendships that are built between residents in the home. Loss of a resident made the other residents reflect on their own mortality, but by far the hardest deaths to deal with were those of the young chronically sick residents, purely due to their age and the impact it had on their friends and families.

There are a few differences between the hospital and nursing home procedures and protocols when the death of a patient or resident occurs. In hospital when the porters are on their way to collect the patient to transfer them to the mortuary, the nursing staff pull the curtains or screens around the beds of all the other patients as a mark of respect and to reduce the potential of distress of seeing that someone had died. In a nursing home, most of the time it was the funeral directors who arrived to transport the deceased to the funeral home. This was unless a sudden or unexpected death occurred, in which case an ambulance would collect them and take them to the hospital mortuary for a post mortem and further investigations. When funeral directors arrived, there was no disguising who they were or what they were there for, as they walked slowly and dutifully through the home in their black uniform suits. Again, as a mark of respect and for privacy the other residents were either returned to their rooms or moved to a communal area away from where the trolley, accompanied by at least two members of funeral staff and a qualified nurse, would pass. Last offices (the preparation of the body) would have been carried out by a qualified nurse and care assistant an hour after the doctor had certified the death. In the case of an expected death there would sometimes would be family members or friends who had been in attendance who would also require support at this time.

If a resident was discovered to have died suddenly, or unexpectedly, for example, while sitting in the communal lounge, which did happen, it was sometimes not immediately noticed by the other residents. In this case a mobile screen would be placed around the resident while the qualified nurse checked the resident and the doctor was called. The other residents would often be moved to another area or returned to their rooms if any kind of waiting period was likely to occur as this helped to avoid upset and speculation. In these cases, if the resident had not been examined or visited by a doctor in the previous three weeks, an ambulance would be requested and the doctor would inform the coroner of the background to the event. Sometimes the police were also informed, depending on the circumstances.

On a happier note, there were sometimes celebrations that required a party to be organised. These included a 100th birthday party, which included the resident receiving a telegram from The Queen. Another special and touching event, during my time at The Carnarvon, was a wedding reception for two of our widowed residents who met and found love in their golden years. They attended a registry office ceremony in Clacton, accompanied by two close family members as witnesses, before returning to the nursing home for a buffet, wedding breakfast prepared by our in-house chef. They were presented with a stunning, two tier wedding cake, made by one of our care assistants, who made celebratory cakes for a part time income. Kim organised for the lounge to be tastefully decorated with flowers for the gathering of close friends, family and the other residents.

The activities coordinator was also responsible for planning and implementing therapeutic activities as part of a guided plan. The most popular of these was reminiscence therapy. One definition of reminiscence therapy states that it involves, "the use of life histories – written, oral, or both – to improve psychological well-being." It is nowadays often used in the care and well-being of older people. This therapeutic activity works by recalling the life and personal experiences of the resident to help them maintain good mental health. The process of reminiscence or recalling events, emotions, places and memories, is thought to improve coping skills, and the research appears to demonstrate positive and lasting results. It is a recognised therapy in the treatment of anxiety, depression, memory loss and dementia.

Residents with dementia often have difficulty remembering what has happened recently, be it events or daily activities, leaving them confused, less confident and vulnerable, but, their long-term memories are often intact. The act of recalling long term memories can be therapeutic and enjoyable. Reminiscence therapy can take place in a group session or on a one-to-one basis and we often found that in a group session, as the residents started to share their individual stories, which are steeped in history and personal experiences, it triggered the memories of others. The act of creating a valuable connection between their past and the present, in an enjoyable and social atmosphere, can lift their spirits and I think it served to improve their self-esteem.

The catchphrase, 'During the war', synonymous and made famous by the television sitcom 'Only Fools and Horses', accurately depicts the way some elderly residents, who lived through or served in WW1 or WW2 whether as children, young adults or service personnel, frequently recalled their many interesting, touching, heart breaking and inspirational stories. Some eagerly shared them at any opportunity, and others were encouraged to do so during reminiscence therapy. I always loved to listen to these stories of wartime experiences. I enjoyed television shows like, 'The Sullivan's' a wartime Australian television soap and others that portrayed the stories of children being sent away to safety as evacuees. I often wondered what that would have felt like from a child's and a parent's perspective.

Elderly people have acquired a wealth of experience, stories and life events which become available to share, and I witnessed that the act of sharing their memories gave them a sense of worth, and reiterated that they had something valuable to contribute. Especially important when sometimes they couldn't recall what they ate at breakfast, but they could recount in detail childhood and wartime experiences!

Fundraising – The Friends of the Carnarvon

The idea of raising funds for residents in a nursing home owned by a national care provider was sometimes misunderstood, but the reality was that the fees charged were for the operational day to day nursing and care provision, the buildings, insurances, food and equipment, etc. The social elements of life, that we can take for granted when we are young and able, like going shopping or on an excursion are luxuries in old age when many rely on the state pension. Therefore, a charitable group was formed within the home, run and administered by the home manager, the activities coordinator and the secretary, all of whom were signatories for the bank account used for the collection and distribution of the cash raised.

The money raised was used for funding trips, theatre tickets, and some small pieces of equipment. We also used the funds to pay for local entertainers to visit the home. These included singers, entertainers and choirs. Their fees were token payments towards their travel and insurance costs and it enabled a full programme of varied entertainment for our residents. The biggest appeal we ran for equipment was for the purchase of our own Graseby pump instead of hiring from the NHS. The methods we used to fundraise included coffee mornings, quiz nights, raffles and prize draws, with prizes donated by local businesses, some of which were also suppliers to the home. These included, the butcher, newsagent, baker and florists. There was a great deal of fun and resident involvement with the fundraising and I believe it gave some of them a sense of purpose. The ones that were able participated in craft afternoons to make items to sell in the foyer or to include as raffle prizes. They enjoyed helping to make posters and selling raffle tickets and relished the opportunity of being able to make a difference to the environment in which they now resided.

Overall, one of the most important effects of this role in the home was that the input of the activities coordinator combined with the management, nursing, care and ancillary staff made the residents feel at home. This enabled them to relax and enjoy life in a safe and caring community. I found so much personal fulfilment in my role and I often took refuge in the nursing home when I was off duty with Samantha, Robert and occasionally with Molly. I felt safe and part of a strong community where everyone looked out for one another. The staff and residents loved having the children there and we would watch television with them, play games or enjoy an evening's entertainment provided by local schools or amateur dramatic groups.

Sarah Jane Butfield

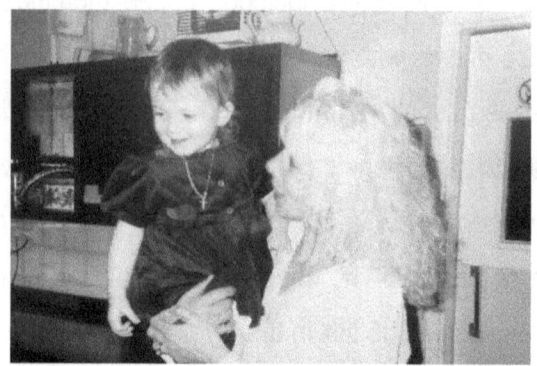

Molly enjoys being centre of attention during quiz night at The Carnarvon.

Chapter Seventeen: The Bill Versus London's Burning!

Advertising and marketing in its many forms was a large part of the strategy, both on a national and local level, in achieving the occupancy levels detailed in that year's business plan. The nursing and residential home business was a highly competitive market place then and premium placement in the relevant publications was considered vital. Of importance were the journals, publications and newspapers that were proven to have a long shelf life or that directly resulted in enquires that converted to resident placements. Advertising space in these media was at a premium and was often booked at least six months or more in advance. Our advertising and marketing budgets were broken down into local and national categories and they were scrutinised and analysed in detail each month during the compilation of the financial variance report with the area manager, and then again quarterly at a national level when the regional, area and home managers met with the executive board members in the London head office.

One of the things that the ANS marketing and promotion department excelled at was supporting the home managers in formulating combined promotional events. These were usually initiated by a home manager, on local level, identifying an event and rallying support from other home managers who would then, as a group, present a proposal for funding to head office. The proposal would detail the expected outcomes, for example, exposure, reach and costs, etc.

The Carnarvon Nursing Home had a standard format of wording for its box adverts that appeared in everything from the local papers to local authority directories which always produced excellent results.

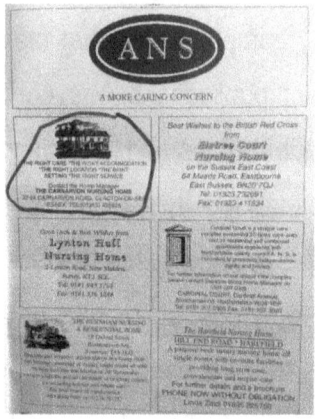

The RIGHT Care

The RIGHT Accommodation

The RIGHT Location

The RIGHT Setting

The RIGHT Service

I always thought it sounded a bit cheesy, but as the old saying goes, 'If it ain't broke don't fix it!'

Bedpans to Boardrooms

One of the biggest joint promotions that I was fortunate to be part of was instigated by me after a telephone call with one of the British Red Cross advertising team whom we had previously advertised with on a local level. They were organising a celebrity football match to be held at Bromley Football Club in Greater London in November as part of the celebrations for the 125th birthday of the British Red Cross, 1870 – 1995 of which Her Royal Highness the Princess of Wales was the patron. The photograph of Princess Diana in the programme was beautiful, however the off the shoulder black dress did little to disguise her prominent shoulder and collarbones. This was during a period when her weight loss was under close scrutiny and made big news after Princess Diana sensationally opened up to the BBC's Martin Bashir, in an interview that she suffered from bulimia. I was an adoring fan of the Princess.

The picture of Princess Diana in the programme

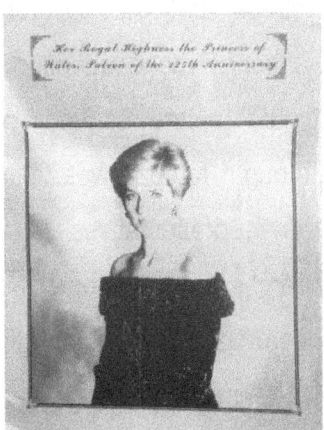

The official programme, priced at £2, for the projected sell out event, would be a glossy souvenir keepsake with a page for autographs. A selection of visitors would have the opportunity to meet the celebrities in a post-match meet and greet session. The teams would consist of cast members from two of my favourite, now iconic, television series of the time; London's Burning and The Bill. Both series were set in the emergency services. I love dramas set in the emergency services or in a hospital setting and even today I cannot get enough of my favourite hospital dramas, Casualty and Holby City for my nursing fix!

As a paid advertiser and supporter of the event we received some complimentary tickets. Although I was not a football fanatic, I was a big fan of the television shows and their cast members so Kim and I took two of the nursing home residents plus Samantha and Robert. A bonus for all of us was being able to meet both teams after the match. I admit to being slightly star-struck, but the children were not and they proceeded to chat to anyone whose attention they could command! Samantha still has her autographed, souvenir copy of the programme and even though she thought football was for boys, she enjoyed the event. There were many representatives from the large variety of organisations and companies that contributed to supporting the event and outside of the boardroom it was my first taste of corporate entertaining as our small team from The Carnarvon were representing ANS. We exchanged business cards and contact details for other joint events and most importantly for the home discussed the option of taking part in a shared waiting list initiative. When it came to fruition this would be a good addition to our strategies for maintaining our occupancy quotas. Another idea spawned from discussions at this event would offer more value to our residents and a potential unique selling point for ANS. Residents would be offered a 'holiday swap' in another home in the ANS group. This would enable them to perhaps incorporate visits to family and friends in other parts of the UK or have a welcome break by the sea. As the Carnarvon Nursing Home occupied a prime position in a popular and historic seaside town we became a popular choice.

The event was a huge success for the British Red Cross. The London's Burning team were extremely popular at the event, I think they had the most young, good looking players! London's Burning, a popular British television action drama programme produced by London Weekend Television aired between 1988 -2002. The dramatic storylines included riots, terrorist plots, domestic and commercial fires and it engaged viewers by portraying the personal and professional lives of members of the London Fire Brigade's Blue Watch, at the fictional Blackwall Fire station.

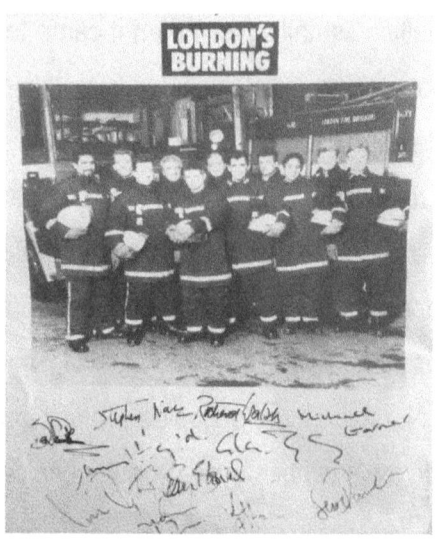

The London's Burning Cast

A couple of the London's Burning stars who took time out to chat to Samantha and Robert included Michael Garner and James Hazeldean. Michael played Geoff Peace, a main character in the shocking episode involving the death of a firefighter for which Geoff would be overcome with guilt. It was aimed at boosting the ratings which were starting to flag. It worked and the series, which I enjoyed, continued successfully for another seven years. James Hazeldine played Bayleaf, the 'mess manager' for the fictitious fire station and was a popular long-term member of the cast.

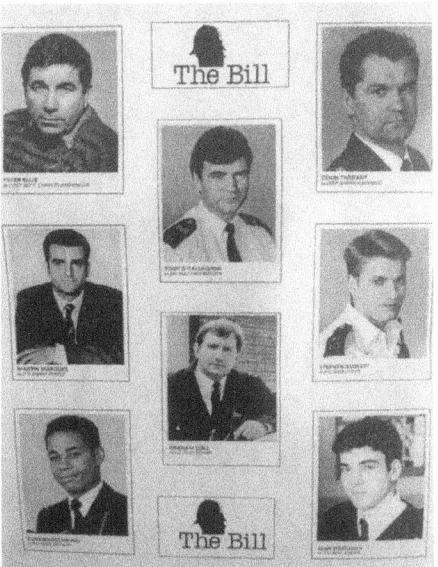

The Bill Cast members

The Bill's team, although sporting more some mature players, were very skilled, I was told. Football was not a sport I knew much about. The Bill was a British police procedural television series, which aired on ITV between 1984 -2010. It was set in a fictional London police station called Sun Hill.

Robert and Samantha both collected the autographs of The Bill's star Graham Cole who played PC Tony Stamp and Eric Richard who played the long-standing desk sergeant Bob Cryer.

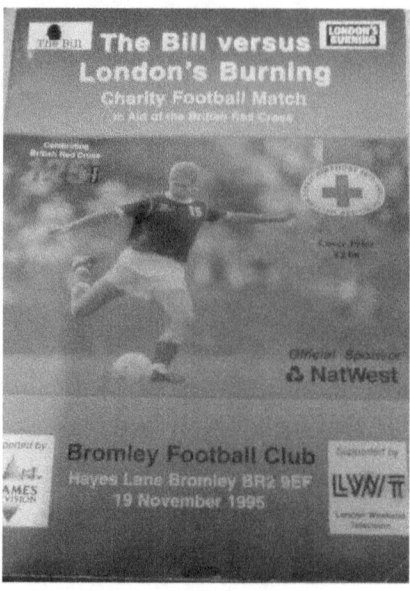

After the event news spread about our involvement with the British Red Cross Celebrations and that we had attended this celebrity event. Samantha's autographed copy of the souvenir program was on display in the foyer for over a month and was a great talking point for new and existing visitors. The residents also loved to show off to their visitors about the high profile we had created, both locally and nationally, and they would collect the newspaper clippings with pride whenever we were reported on.

The Carnarvon as a nursing home, and myself as the manager, attracted some local media attention following this event and I was more than a little flattered and slightly red faced when at the next head office boardroom meeting I was given a special mention as the 'most creative, rookie manager' they had ever worked with!' They said that, "I had a creative flare and an innovative streak not usually found in clinical nurses and that they intended to nurture the talent they had spotted." I liked the sound of that and I felt proud that, despite the events in my personal life, I was not only maintaining my career but potentially growing it against the odds.

Within a few weeks, it was Christmas. I planned to spend it at The Carnarvon with Samantha and Robert so that they were surrounded by people and fun events to distract them from the fact that it would be a Christmas without Molly. The staff and residents had a wonderful time, as did the children.

Christmas at The Carnarvon.

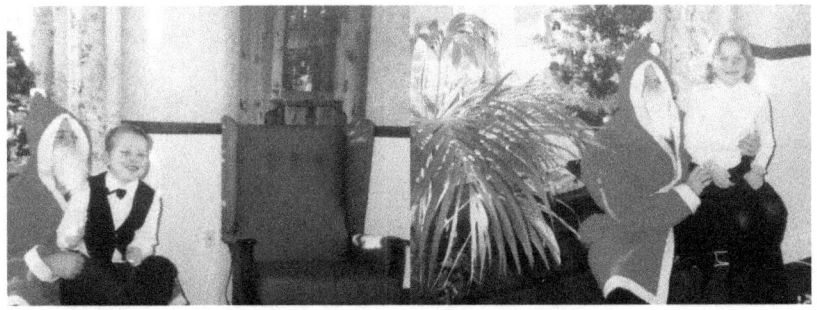

Samantha and Robert meet Father Christmas at The Carnarvon on Christmas Day

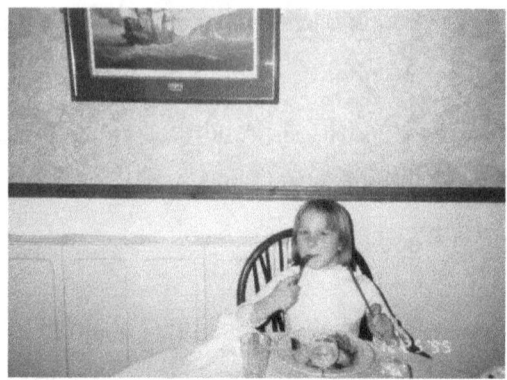

Samantha enjoys Christmas lunch with the residents.

Chapter Eighteen: The beginning of the end

At work, I was the 'go to' person for the nursing home staff, residents and visitors. The one that would help them with problems and concerns or whom they could approach for advice and support. From the moment that I put my work uniform blouse on and applied my make-up, I became that person. I hid behind that uniform during the day and it enabled me to function as a human being. The only personal reassurance that I could give myself was that I thought I was doing 'alright.' At this point, as a nurse and mum, the fact was that I was providing for myself and my children. We had a home, food, friends and family. Despite this, the emptiness, guilt and desperation I felt, in relation to the way I had allowed myself to be used and manipulated including losing full time care of my baby girl, ate away at my heart. When I didn't keep myself busy, and distracted with work or the children, I would drift into a state of despair and would find myself crawling into bed at 7pm as soon as Samantha and Robert were asleep, begging for the day to be over. I didn't recognise the signs of the depressive state into which I had slipped until Lynnette called round one evening. It was 7.30pm and I sleepily answered the door in my pyjamas.

"Why are all the lights out?"

"I was in bed."

"In bed! At this time? Where are the kids?"

"They are in bed."

Well they had been. Now they were both poking their heads around the stair bannisters to see who I was talking to in the hallway below.

"It's OK kids, pop back to bed, I am just going to have a chat with mummy." Lynnette reassured them.

Grabbing me by the arm Lynnette dragged me into the lounge, pushing me backwards into the armchair.

"Now look here, enough is enough. We are going to sort this out once and for all. What are you doing with your life? You have a great job, wonderful kids and yet you let that idiot rule your every thought and movement by dangling the carrot of a few hours with Molly. This must stop!"

I knew she was right, but she didn't understand. She wasn't a mum and I truly felt like I was the only person in the world that this had ever happened to. How could anyone understand the pain I felt. At this point, my little girl was growing up with her dad and his new fiancé, well actually his cousin from Australia, but let's not go there! Despite all the money I had thrown at legal advice and proceedings and even trying to bribe Jack at one point, my efforts had been in vain. He worked the system, living on social security benefits, obtaining free legal advice and emotionally he pushed me around because he knew he could. All he had to do was threaten me with, "You'll never see her again," and I did as I was told.

I was now crying, something which still came easily to me every day, at least once, but tonight it was different, it was like a pipe had burst. My eyes, nose and mouth were awash. I think I may well have drowned if Lynnette had not roughly wiped my whole face with a tea towel. She put her arms around me and held me so tight that momentarily it felt like my world stopped, everything was quiet except for me trying to catch my breath through the tears.

Lynnette looked me in the eye and was silent. Then she drew back, "Oh my god Sarah I know what you've done!"

My eyes were drawn to looking at the floor as I desperately wanted to avoid her gaze. She lifted my chin forcing my face upwards and as the tears fell I will never forget the look of disgust in her eyes.

"Tell me I'm wrong, please tell me that, or tell me something."

She wasn't wrong, she had been the one person I dreaded telling what I had done and now that moment had passed, she knew me so well she had guessed. She would never understand, no one would, and I was so ashamed I hadn't even admitted to myself the gravity of my actions.

I was pregnant with another child of Jack's.

I know what you are thinking now, how could she? Why would she? etc., etc. And yes, if I was on the outside and someone was telling me this, I would be thinking exactly the same, and more. But I was on the inside, and I needed my daughter and when, during a visit with Molly, Jack started to talk about the chance of a reconciliation, I grabbed it. As always it was not what it appeared, it was a means to borrow money for a car, but now I was carrying his child. With hormones surging, and in denial, the very last thing I wanted or needed was for anyone else to know.

"So, what now?" The words were ringing loudly in my ears as Lynnette withdrew and flung herself on the sofa. "Are you keeping it?"

The reality was that it had not, at any point, crossed my mind not to keep the baby. Was that an option? Could I have an abortion? No, I couldn't – I knew that for a fact and that was probably why the thought had never entered my head.

"Yes, I'm keeping it."

"And how exactly, will you manage that?" Lynnette's tone was indignant and momentarily I felt threatened by her. "Do you know what

Sarah, I don't think I know you at all. After everything he has put you and the kids through and you have turned into nothing less than his whore. I'm leaving. I can't talk to you right now."

With that said she was gone, and I was alone. As the front door slammed shut a flurry of arms and legs was suddenly crawling over me as Samantha and Robert ran into the room and jumped on my lap. They were hugging me and Samantha said, "We love you mummy." With tears still flowing I kissed them both. The bond we had would give me the strength to get through whatever the world would throw at me now, but one thing was for sure I would not be giving up another baby to Jack or to anyone else. If ever I have had an excuse or a reason to label myself as a failure or a victim it would have been during this period as the list of compromises and sacrifices I made grew, as did the number of people I hurt by shutting them out due to my shame.

Over the next few months I had some difficult decisions to make as I kept the news of my pregnancy under wraps. I managed to conceal it until I was six months pregnant and I deliberately distanced myself from people at work as I knew the gossip had already started. 'Who was the father? Is it Jack's? Will Sarah be leaving?' The residents were so lovely when they found out. By his time, I had made some wonderful friendships and some of them were like adoptive parents and grandparents to me and the children. I could not share with anyone what I had done, but it didn't take much for them to start trying to piece it all together and elaborate on it until it resembled a storyline worthy of a television soap drama.

When Jack found out about the baby, he said something along the line of, "If you thought getting pregnant would make me come back to you think again. A thirty something with three kids, who would want that?"

That actually was a relief because the last thing I wanted was him back. I only ever wanted Molly. The hardest part involved telling ANS that I was pregnant and going on maternity leave within a few weeks. Later, having to tell them that I would not be able to return as the home manager broke my heart, but I would not be leaving my new baby with anyone ever and so working there would be out of the equation. The beginning of my illustrious career with ANS was now ending, but what lay ahead? Was this the end of my nursing career? I hoped not, but for now it was family first.

Jaime Lee was born on 12th September 1996.

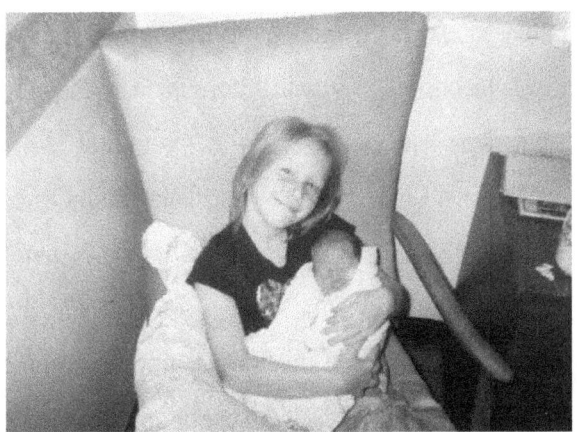

Sibling love:
Samantha proudly holds her new-born baby sister Jaime Lee in SCBU

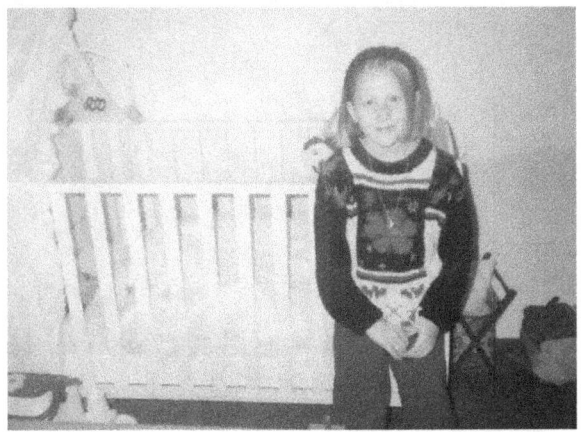

Jaime arrives home from hospital and Samantha is my helping hand with a new baby in the house.

Although Jack had no interest in Jaime, he visited and hung around the house on a daily basis, as if trying to deter other visitors, which was effective as no one liked him. Even my small circle of true friends and family would drive past without stopping if they saw his car outside. Jack would bring Molly with him, which made me happy, so I didn't turn them away. He would come in, handover Molly, then go to sleep on the sofa, which was fine. We had little to say to one another. I took every opportunity to spend even just a few minutes with my beautiful little girl who, at two and half years old, with her big brown eyes, made my heart melt. I had missed so many memorable moments and events in her short life to date and every small period of time spent with her was precious so I grabbed it shamelessly.

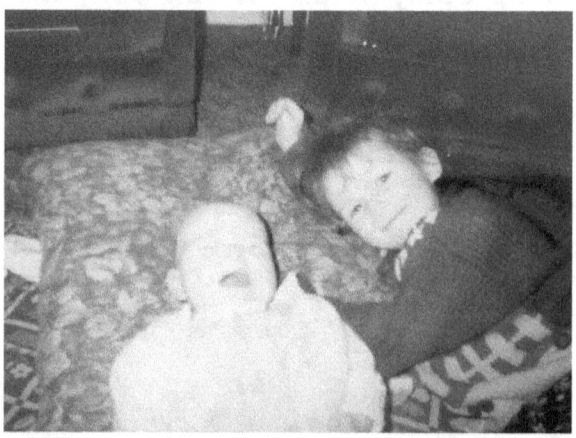

Molly and her baby sister Jaime Lee

For a few months after Jaime was born Jack started letting Molly stay with me more often and for longer. Samantha and Robert loved this and I enjoyed times with all four of my children together. I would later find out this supposedly generous act of allowing me more time with Molly was because his latest 'girlfriend' had a busy social life that he was trying to integrate and having a small child in tow didn't help him on this occasion.

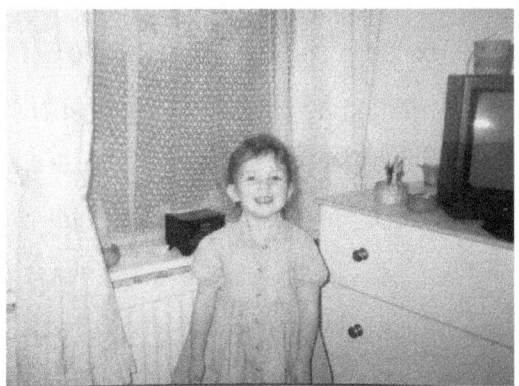

Molly poses for Samantha during a weekend stay.

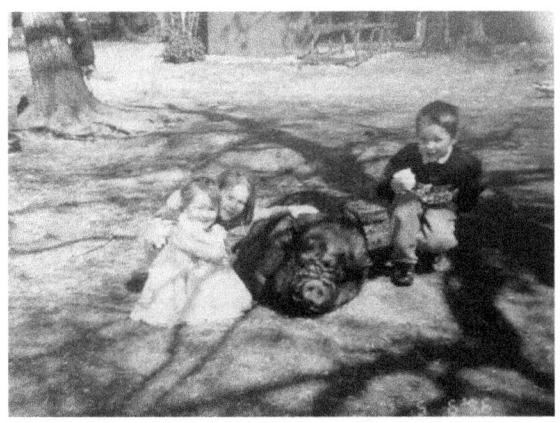

Family time Samantha, Robert and Molly

Now, as an unemployed nurse, and single mum, I needed to find ways to earn a living, but I still could not contemplate leaving Jaime. I started child-minding for a local family five days a week as they both worked full time as accountants and commuted to London. Their little boy, Asnee, was only three and not yet old enough for full time nursery school. This worked well and I also managed to find a couple of cleaning jobs where I could take Jaime with me on the weekends when Samantha and Robert went to spend time with Keith. I was determined to provide for my family and I was sad that it couldn't be by pursuing the career I loved, but there seemed to be no way of achieving that.

Lynnette eventually forgave me for keeping the truth from her, and as the valued friend that she was, one of the first things she did when Jaime was about six months old was to persuade me to book in for a tubal sterilisation at the Marie Curie clinic. I knew this was for the best and I only agreed to go if she cared for Jaime whilst I was there. She knew how vulnerable I could be and so she visited at least three times a week, if not daily. Jack hated her and now the roles were reversed and he drove past when he saw her car parked outside.

Not working as a nurse, in any role, and the loss of my self-respect, self-confidence and dignity was a big price to pay, but would it be worth it? Could I hold my little family together and find a degree of happiness to ease even just a small part of the pain I suffered?

Was this the end of the line for my nursing career?

Find out in book three! You can take a sneak preview of the start of chapter one at the end of this book.

Sarah Jane Butfield

Epilogue Written by Shontae Brewster

What ever happened to the fun-loving girl who almost by accident entered the world of nursing after leaving school?

She went on to become an accomplished and valued nurse, rapidly gaining nursing and management experience in the aged care sector whilst growing her family and dealing with personal challenges and tragedies. What we also know, and what I personally admire about Sarah Jane, is that her brutally honest approach to sharing the dark and sometimes seemingly impossible life challenging events can depict her as weak, however she always finds a way to pull herself and her precious family back to the surface to move on in the search of 'better things to come'. I think it is her faith and total belief that there is always something better waiting to happen that demonstrates her positive approach to challenges and as she matures and becomes stronger on the back of adversity this personal trait is growing. Sarah Jane doesn't see it in herself in these early books, but those who she helps and cares about regularly remind her to 'take some of her own advice' and later she will!

Some of the many unanswered questions while we wait for the next book in The Nomadic Nurse series involve contemplating what Sarah Jane did next and where?

How would Sarah Jane get her nursing career back on track now that she was a single mother of four with a baby, a part time toddler and two school aged children?

Could she protect Samantha, Robert and Jaime from a traumatised childhood as her legal and personal battles with Jack ensue?

Would she win custody or regular contact with her daughter Molly and have a chance of a close mother daughter relationship?

All of this and more will be answered as we find Sarah Jane pursuing a new career pathway in a new location in book three. To get a sneak peek of the start of the of the opening chapter keep reading to the end of this book.

A quote from my review:

"A true story of survival entwined in an intriguing and diverse nursing memoir depicting Sarah Jane's professional and personal journey from Bedpans to Boardrooms."

Appendix I: Glossary of Medical Terms and Abbreviations

COPD Chronic Obstructive Pulmonary Disease is a group of progressive lung diseases. The most common are emphysema and chronic bronchitis.

Oncology: a branch of medicine that deals with the prevention, diagnosis and treatment of cancer.

EMI (Elderly, Mentally, Impaired, formerly infirm)

IIP (Investors in People) Awards

NHS (National Health Service)

QA (Quality Assurance)

RGN (Registered General Nurse)

RMN (Registered Mental Nurse)

SRN (State Registered Nurse)

YCS (Young Chronically Sick)

Appendix II: Reference links

Pastoral Care

https://www.questia.com/library/journal/1P3-2404917771/defining-pastoral-care-for-older-people-in-residential

Legislation for YCS

1970 The Chronically Sick and Disabled Persons Act

http://www.legislation.gov.uk/ukpga/1970/44/section/1

PEG feeding

http://patient.info/doctor/peg-feeding-tubes-indications-and-management

Sarah Jane Butfield

Sneak preview of Book 3! What a mess I've made!

Who would have thought that a seemingly intelligent, professionally qualified woman could have allowed herself and her life to become unravelled at the hands of an Essex wide boy and would be Casanova. 'Hook, line and sinker', as the saying goes, was how I had become trapped and ensnared in Jack's web of lies, deceit and unscrupulous behaviour. I knew something had to change, not only for my own sanity and health, but for the protection of my children. However, I was too scared and lacked the self-confidence to even consider acting. Here I was, a 31-year mother of four young children, living on a low wage for child-minding and cleaning for a local Asian family, topped up by child benefit and housing benefit. Where was my beloved career I that I had worked so hard to achieve and sacrificed my marriage for now?

Why had I let a man destroy everything I had fought for? Had my sacrifices to carve out a career over the years been for nothing? Could I pull my now seemingly worthless existence back from the brink? Over dramatic? Possibly. But to be honest it was only my children that prevented me from ending my life to escape the hellish situation I now found myself in. Having always been a believer in fate and that, 'everything happens for a reason', I had convinced myself by this point that I deserved everything that was now being thrown at me. Karma was paying me back for being weak-willed in the early days of meeting Jack. That said, I cannot regret our fateful meeting or the two wonderful children we conceived as that would be a far greater sin and something I could never forgive myself for.

At this time, I had only one true friend, Lynnette. She was a fellow Registered Nurse whom I had worked with at The Carnarvon Nursing Home and who was a great listener. As a fiery redhead, she also did not hold back on sharing her opinion on some of my life choices, especially those connected to Jack.

I now know that, as passive observers, Lynnette and others could see the devastation unfolding, and my inability or unwillingness to stop it. Lynnette's partner Richard was a fire fighter in Colchester and they were both career orientated with no desire to start a family. However, they enjoyed a pseudo family with me and my young children coming as friend's package. Living as a single mum at the time, I didn't go out, despite their numerous offers to babysit. They constantly encouraged me to meet new people even by resorting to the personal ads in the local newspaper because after all, 'you have to start somewhere Sarah'. Despite declining gracefully and wanting to be alone they would instead turn up at around 7.30pm when the kids were in bed armed with a bottle of wine and a Blockbuster rented video.

One evening they arrived and Lynnette said, "Right, enough is enough! Get changed we are going out, Richard will babysit. A cab will be here in 20 minutes."

We all know not to argue with redheads, I have two redheaded sisters' and have learned to my cost over the years not to cross them. I ran upstairs, changed out of my fluffy pyjamas and into a dress. Lynnette stood in the bedroom doorway with her hands on her hips.

"We are not going to the pub with you dressed like you are going to the Women's Institute. Where did you even get that 50s style mummy dress?"

I was taken aback, but quickly removed it and grabbed my jeans and a silky blouse. Holding it high above my head on the hanger, I said, "Is this better?"

"It will do, but we really need to go clothes shopping – soon!"

As I put the silky blouse on I realised that I hadn't worn it for over three years and, having had a baby since then, let's just say my bust was a bit bigger and the blouse a lot tighter! With no time to waste and few other clothes to choose from I headed for the bathroom. Standing in front of the mirror with an overflowing laundry basket behind me and nappy buckets in the bath I felt distinctly overdressed and uncomfortable after many months of wearing little make-up, jeans and tee-shirts or my pyjamas. I brushed my hair and scooped it back with a black plastic Alice band. I applied some black mascara and turned to walk downstairs. Lynnette was there again.

"Good god girl, at least put some lippy on!" She was armed with a handful of lipsticks all of which looked far too bright and garish for a trip to the pub. I took what looked like the least sparkling option and applied a thin layer quickly blotting it with some toilet paper. A car horn sounded.

"That's the taxi – where are your shoes?" Lynnette shouted, not realising I was close behind her.

Shoes? I didn't think my trusty trainers would be suitable for this excursion so I grabbed my black knee high boots and ran downstairs.

"Well, well, well!" said Richard, "If that's what happens in under twenty minutes then Colchester had better watch out if we give you more notice next time!"

Lynnette thrust my denim jacket into my arms and I grabbed my purse from the dresser. As I walked down the hall towards the front door, which was already wide open, I glanced in the mirror and momentarily didn't recognise myself. I got into the back seat of the taxi and continued zipping up my boots. I looked forward at the driver and immediately noticed the striking resemblance he bore to Richard. I looked across at

Lynnette about to comment on this and noticed she was getting out of the car. I reached to open my door.

"Stop! Don't even think about it. You and Nigel are going to the pub." Hardly pausing for breath she continued, "Sarah, this is Nigel, Richard's brother; Nigel, this is Sarah my good friend who is long overdue a night out."

I felt like a charity case and could feel tears welling up in my eyes. It was like those awkward teenage years all over again. You are overcome by embarrassment and just want to run and hide as you feel your face flush brighter than the lipstick you are wearing.

"Oh, and Sarah don't worry, he has relationship baggage as well so you two will get on just fine."

Lynnette was referring to another of my regular excuses for not wanting to enter another relationship, because I have too many kids and too much baggage for anyone to risk getting involved with me. Lynnette slammed the car door shut and I watched as the front door to my house closed as she returned inside.

Nigel, who was now turned in his seat looking straight at me said, "OK then, where shall we go?" I was still in shock.

"Oh, I don't know any of the pubs around here you choose."

We drove in silence for a few minutes and then both tried to speak at the same time to break the deafening silence that existed despite the radio playing Duran Duran in the background.

"Did you know about this?"

"As if! I am still trying to work out why I agreed to do a cab job on my night off – family can be persuasive, hey?"

We arrive and walked into the pub which thankfully was quiet. Nigel ordered our drinks and we settled ourselves at a small table near an open fire with a leather chair on either side. Momentarily I forgot that we were in a pub as we fell deep into conversation as if we had known each other for years. The noise of the pub as its custom increased was white noise in the background to which I soon became oblivious.

It soon became obvious that we had more in common than just both being separate or divorced with children that we loved. We both had an affinity with Cornwall, having holidayed there as kids or in early adulthood. We loved 80s music and enjoyed camping. The more we talked, the more we discovered about the similarities in our lives, both past and present. Even to the point of discovering that I was in the same post-natal ward as his ex-wife when I gave birth to Molly. Nigel's daughter Clair was born on the same ward days earlier. How eerie was that? Actually, I found it slightly disturbing for some reason!

Did this all mean something? Two slightly damaged people with a love of family and outdoor pursuits meet on a blind date set up by a best friend and her partner. Would this be a match made in heaven?

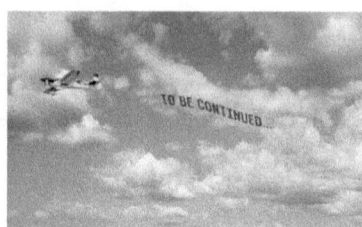

In book three find out how Sarah Jane attempts to get her career back on track with a new qualification and an unexpected career pathway which leads her into the world of nursing agencies.

About the author, Sarah Jane Butfield

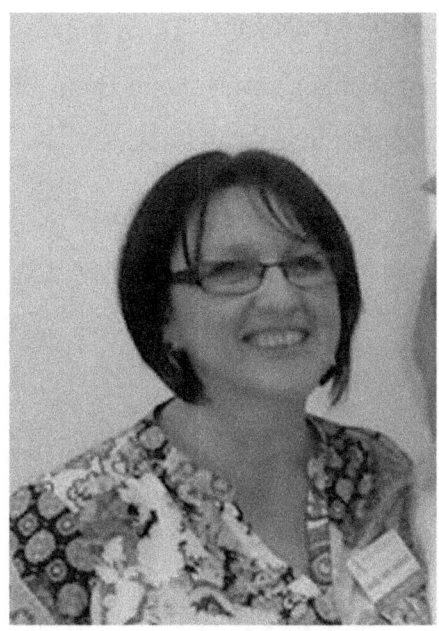

Sarah Jane Butfield, CEO at Rukia Publishing, is also an international best-selling author in her own right. She carefully and professionally combines these positions with her family roles of wife, mother and grandmother. After a successful career as a Registered General Nurse, spanning 28 years, Sarah Jane has a reputation for caring, and being 'a people person'. Now as an established, and respected memoirist, she shares her honest, touching life experiences in her travel and nursing memoir series'. She hopes to inspire and motivate her readers to 'always believe there is something better ahead.'

Sarah Jane lives in South Wales with her husband, Nigel, and their two playful Australian Cattle dogs, Dave and Buster. She is a proud mother and step-mother to her seven strong 'Brady Bunch', and she loves every minute of their convoluted lives.

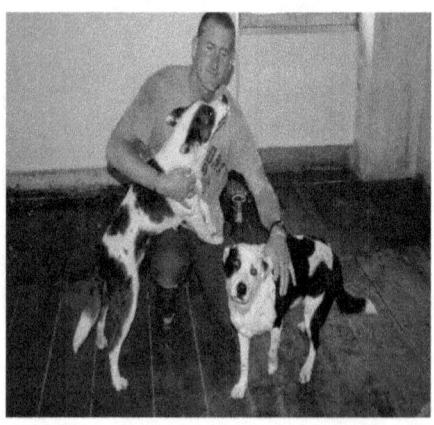

Nigel with Dave and Buster

Keep in touch!

Sarah Jane loves to interact with her readers so feel free to connect on social media:

Twitter @SarahJanewrites

Facebook:

www.facebook.com/AuthorSarahJaneButfield
www.facebook.com/Twodogsandasuitcase
www.facebook.com/OurFrugalSummerinCharente
www.facebook.com/Ooh-Matron-1646665865549530/timeline/

Sarah Jane Butfield

We Love Memoirs

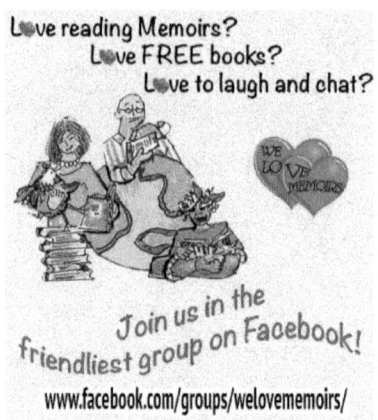

If you love memoirs, why not join Sarah Jane and over 3000 memoirs readers and authors at:

www.facebook.com/groups/welovememoirs/

Be sure to say Sarah Jane sent you!

Travel Memoirs by Sarah Jane Butfield

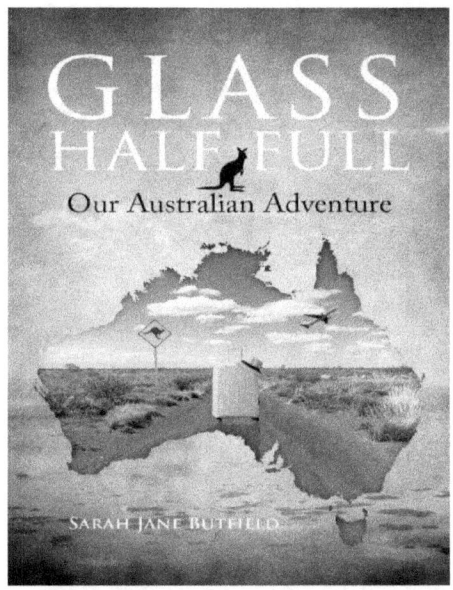

Glass Half Full: Our Australian Adventure

Striving to keep their Glass Half Full, this expat family struggle to cope with loss and grieving, Post-Traumatic Stress Disorder and the devastating Brisbane floods. Life is never without its challenges, but how many life-changing events can one family endure before they reach breaking point?

Find out in this heart wrenching and touching true story. After enduring divorce and numerous child custody battles, Sarah Jane knew that moving to Australia was their only chance of future happiness and that as a family they were making the right decisions. Living the Australian dream in Alice Springs was everything they hoped for until life-changing events started to test the foundations of this resilient family. Using every ounce of positive thinking they could muster, they struggled on. However, just as they thought the worst was over Mother Nature intervened and washed away the roots to their new life during the Brisbane floods of 2011. This story lets you experience Australian life with an inspirational woman and her courageous family, as they struggle to survive challenging life events and keep their dreams alive.

Here's what readers are saying about Glass Half Full: Our Australian Adventure.

"An incredibly well-written book, full of emotion, and very descriptive. I feel I have travelled this journey with Sarah and her family."

"Sometimes the author made me feel so close to her situations by her brilliant descriptions that I almost felt I had witnessed it first-hand. Very clever writing."

"It is amazing what people can withstand and still move forward. Their youngest was on a great adventure. As life gets in the way of happiness this couple keeps picking themselves up and moving forward. A must read for those intending to take up life in Australia or Tasmania."

"With vivid descriptions of people and places, this riveting story is about a family who leave England for a better life in Australia. They carefully plan each step of their long-term goals; to get permanent residency in Australia, become financially secure, and maintain a happy and healthy relationship with their large and scattered family. Glass Half Full, our Australian adventure. Everything goes as planned until a sequence of life-changing events stops them in their tracks, and then mother nature devastates their

carefully laid out master plan. An amazing journey of people living life to its fullest. Inspirational!"

books2read.com/GlassHalfFull

Two Dogs and a Suitcase: Clueless in Charente

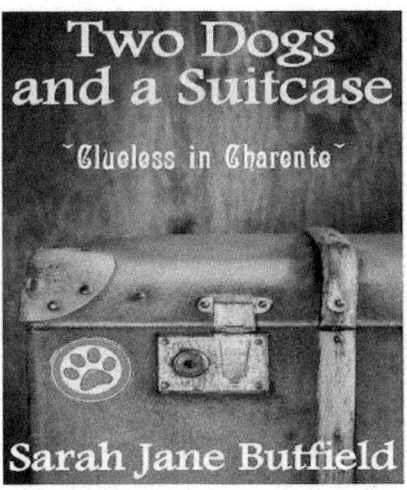

The title says it all: what we have and where we are. This book, the sequel to Glass Half Full: Our Australian Adventure, follows our French exploits as we endeavour to rebuild our lives in another new country, after spending four and half years in Australia. Our goal, or hope for the immediate future, is to focus positively on the present, so that we can start a new, optimistic future back in Europe. Our main aim is to be nearer to the children, leaving the dark clouds of the challenges we faced in Australia as a distant memory. Journey with us as we arrive in rural South West France; enjoy my reflections, thoughts, and observations about my family, our new surroundings, and our lifestyle. Follow the journey of my writing career and how we start our renovation project while managing our convoluted family life. Once again, we will laugh, cry, and enjoy life to the fullest with a generous helping of positive spin thrown in for good measure.

Read our story….books2read.com/TwoDogs

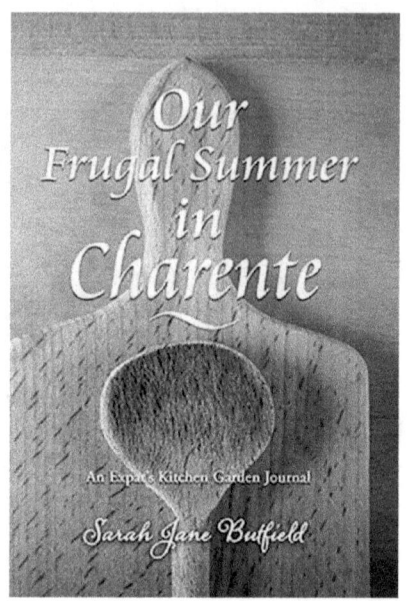

NEW SECOND EDITION - OCTOBER 2016

Our Frugal Summer in Charente: An Expat's Kitchen Garden Journal - nominated as one of the 'Top 50 Self-Published Books Worth Reading' in the Read Freely Awards 2015.

Reader Review quote:

"5 stars for Our frugal summer. I am a foodie!! I loved this book inciting her frugal lifestyle, with superb recipes and life in Charente. a must read. by Angela."

Meet Sarah Jane, a woman with a reputation for culinary catastrophe who tries to keep her family fed in challenging circumstances in rural France. Frugal living was not part of the plan when they arrived from Australia to undertake the renovation of a quaint cottage in the Charente. However, when life throws them a curve-ball the challenge was set. How to survive in France with very little money and two Australian cattle dogs. The answer came in the form of 5 chickens, 4 ducks and a vegetable garden! The frugal plan was to save money by any means possible, to enable any money they could earn to be invested into continuing the renovation of the cottage. In true 'Good Life' style Sarah Jane attacks this challenge head on by keeping some small livestock and converting a garden, that resembled a meadow, into a French 'potager' or kitchen garden. The French tradition of using produce from their 'potagers' is renowned for enabling families to create meals that are healthy, cost effective and simple.

There are 31 recipes for a variety of food and drinks, included in a month by month account, of how they transformed a neglected garden into a frugal yet productive expat kitchen garden.

Book club members say:

"Sarah has a wonderful writing style and a lively sense of humour and the subject matter of this book was an entertaining and interesting change. This author has taken me out of my comfort zone nationwide and I'm so glad she did. Try it you will love it." Reviewer -swnseajac

Sarah Jane Butfield

"The great thing about this particular book is that it is about forgetting what we don't have, and taking instead what we do, and making the most of it. This is a principle the author seems to apply to her life, also and that comes across clearly in the memoir sections." Reviewer – Margaret

Available at all good online bookstores here:

books2read.com/ourfrugalsummer

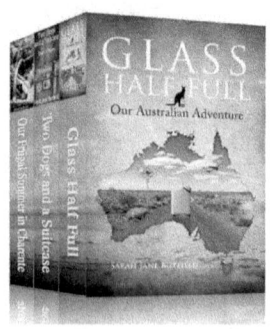

Also available as a boxset books2read.com/MemoirBoxset

Other Books by Sarah Jane Butfield

What, Why, Where, When, Who & How Book Promotion Series

All links available on www.sarahjanebutfield.com

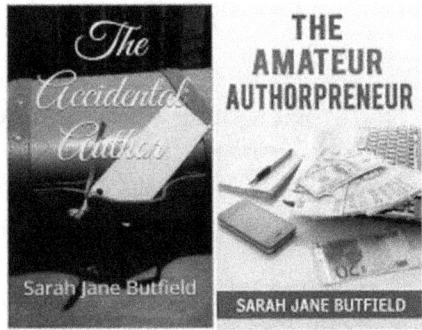

The Accidental Author

Permanently FREE

This is book 1 in a new series which looks at self-publishing for beginners and the skills needed for ongoing book marketing and promotion. This e-books series is based on the experiences of author Sarah Jane Butfield who writes travel memoirs, non-fiction books and romance short stories.

The Accidental Author introduces the author and this series of self-help e-books for new or aspiring self-published authors. The introduction starts with how and why Sarah Jane came to write and self-publish Glass Half Full: Our Australian Adventure. Find out how an aspiring author aims to be discovered while learning on the job how to write, publish and launch a new career in writing.

"Sarah Jane's never give up approach to life and anything she turns her hand to is beyond admirable." John Roberts

"A must read for any aspiring author or readers interested in the life of a self-published author. Sarah Jane's never give up approach to life and anything she turns her hand to is beyond admirable."

Book 2 The Amateur Authorpreneur

The Amateur Authorpreneur is a beginners' guide for authors who intend to develop their writing into a business, addressing the important task of book promotion and marketing. We look at laying the foundations of the authorpreneur book promotion toolkit, building a fan base on social media and much more.

You've written a book or you plan to - what do you need to consider?

What does it offer readers?

Why will they buy it?

Where are your readers?

When will you publish it?

Who are you?

How do you promote it!

Find out how to take the business of being an author up a gear to become an authorpreneur. The Amateur Authorpreneur will describe, using the What, Why Where, When, Who & How template, the process of taking the first steps into combining the craft of being an author with the business of marketing your work. Here are some beta reader comments:

"Aspiring authors will feel reassured that whatever their age or IT ability all of the skills needed to become an authorpreneur are achievable."

A non-author beta reader said, "I have discovered skills and tips that now helps me in both my personal and professional social media interactions."

"An avid reader who enjoys the work of indie authors was, "amazed at what's involved behind the scenes."

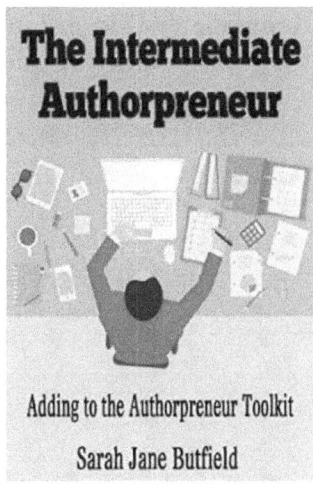

Book 3 The Intermediate Authorpreneur

Sarah Jane Butfield

Reader feedback:

"This guide is just what I needed to set my goals for the future"

"I am awe of what an indie author has to know and do on a daily basis, as a reader I applaud you all."

"A valuable guide and essential reading for all new authors or those that need to refocus their social media presence"

"The evidence based graphs and statistics were a nice, reassuring touch. Sarah definitely keeps it real."

Find out how to get your writing business started in easy to follow, simple steps which breaks down the fears and myths of social media and networking for aspiring and new authors. It's not rocket science and anyone can do it! Get started today and feel free to network with the author for additional support on your book marketing and promotional journey.

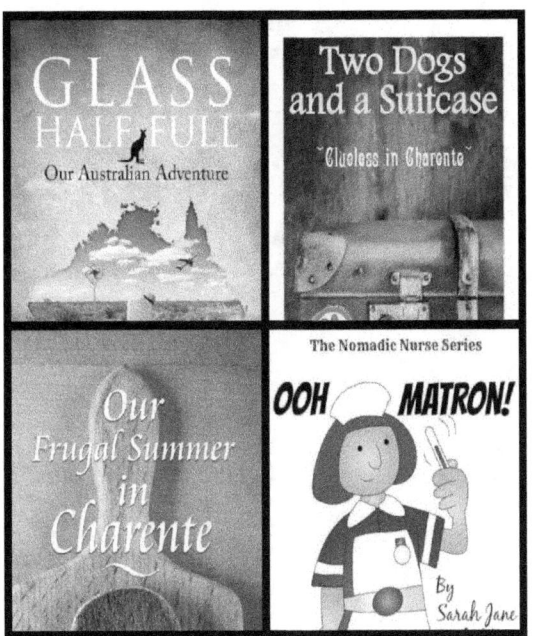

To hear about my latest books first, sign up for my exclusive mailing list. (No spam ever, I promise.)

http://eepurl.com/0IuML

Thank you for reading.

Sarah Jane Butfield

www.ingramcontent.com/pod-product-compliance
Lightning Source LLC
Chambersburg PA
CBHW071421180526
45170CB00001B/177